CW00796204

Psychopharmacology for Health Professionals

DATE DUE

GAYLORD

PRINTED IN U.S.A.

DEDICATION

For our children

Nathan Usher

Melissa & Kyle Boyle

Kieran Barber

Psychopharmacology for Health Professionals

Kim Usher
Kim Foster
Shane Bullock

ELSEVIER

Mosby
is an imprint of Elsevier

Elsevier Australia. ACN 001 002 357
(a division of Reed International Books Australia Pty Ltd)
Tower 1, 475 Victoria Avenue, Chatswood, NSW 2067

National Library of Australia Cataloguing-in-Publication Data

Usher, Kim.

Psychopharmacology for health professionals /
Kim Usher, Kim Foster, Shane Bullock.

ISBN: 978 0 7295 3860 2 (pbk.)

Includes index.
Bibliography.

Psychopharmacology.
Psychotropic drugs.

Foster, Kim.
Bullock, Shane.

615.78

Publishing Editor: Luisa Cecotti
Developmental Editor: Sabrina Chew
Publishing Services Manager: Helena Klijn
Editorial Coordinator: Lauren Allsop
Edited by Linda Littlemore
Proofread by Tim Learner
Index by Max McMaster
Cover design by Avril Makula
Internal design and typesetting by Pindar New Zealand
Printed in Australia by Ligare

CONTENTS

FOREWORD

This is a concise, yet comprehensive psychopharmacology textbook written for the range of health professionals in Australia and New Zealand who care for consumers with mental illness in our communities. The text is easy to read and there is good use of diagrams, tables and boxes that hold the reader's attention. The information is well supported by the literature and is up-to-date.

The text sets the scene well and Chapter 2 provides an overview of the neuroscience of the brain that gives the student an excellent understanding of the mechanisms of action of psychotropics. This is unusual in similar texts. The book also takes a novel but appropriate approach to presentation of the material in the chapters that cover the psychopathologies pertinent to a group of medications, rather than adherence to a specific diagnostic approach. Thus, medication used for disturbance of cognition and perception includes the major psychoses as well as dementias.

Kim Usher and colleagues have written in my view an almost unique text, in that there is a thorough attempt to present an appreciation of what is involved in taking (and being given involuntarily) medications from the perspective of consumers and carers. This is refreshing and adds important information to help guide practitioners. In addition, the sections on the use of medications in Indigenous peoples (Ch 7) and on PRN medication (Ch 8) also provide an understanding that is seldom to be found in other books.

Students and their educators will appreciate the reflective tasks and teaching and learning activities. These focus the reader and, if undertaken with thoughtfulness and diligence, will help both in formal assessment but, more importantly, in improving consumer–clinician interaction, clinical skills and prescribing practices.

This text is appropriate for students of psychology, nursing and social work, as well as medical undergraduates, family medicine post-graduates, and allied health professionals involved in the care of those with mental illness. It is engaging, based on sound science and provides important insights from consumers and carers.

Professor Phillipa Hay
Foundation Chair of Mental Health
School of Medicine, University of Western Sydney

PREFACE

In contrast to many of the standard books and texts on psychotropic medications that tend to offer lists of medications, their actions, side effects and indications based primarily on the assumptions of the scientific approach, in this text we aim to offer a more comprehensive perspective that recognises the many stakeholder perspectives involved in the prescribing, taking and administering of these medications.

The text has been designed to be interactive and to engage you as the reader. By interactive, we mean the sharing of information based on the best available evidence and our own experience, as well as the personal experience of consumers who have used psychotropic medications and the experience of health professionals who administer them and work with consumers taking psychotropic medications. Each of these perspectives provides information that, when combined, can give a more comprehensive and inclusive understanding of the usage of psychotropic medications. At the same time, we encourage you as the reader to engage with the information you are reading and explore it critically, using it to inform and extend your understanding and clinical practice. Throughout the text, we have included thinking challenges, chat boxes, clinical alert boxes and relevant tables, figures and diagrams to provide you with opportunities to reflect upon and analyse the many aspects of psychotropic medication usage. At the end of each chapter we have identified useful websites and resources and provided direction to useful further reading related to the topic. As you work through each chapter, we encourage you to maintain a critical awareness of the information you read, in order to expand and develop your own views and perspectives on this group of treatments.

We have also taken a fresh approach to discussion of the major groups of psychotropic medications. You will note that in each chapter we have referred to groups of medications to treat major features of mental disorder, such as cognition and perception, affect, anxiety and sleep, and we have also included a chapter on substance use, in preference to the more traditional reference to particular groups of disorder such as schizophrenia or mood/affective disorders. This approach is based on our shared understandings and experience of the medical/scientific approach to diagnosis and treatment of mental disorders currently used in most Western countries including Australia and New Zealand. Our perspective on mental illness is based on understanding the person as being distinct from their illness, and knowing that language is important in understanding attitudes towards mental illness and disorders. In this book, while we describe mental disorders, we focus more on the symptoms and features of them. As a result, Chapters 3 to 6 only provide an overview of disorders; for a more comprehensive account of each mental health disorder, the reader is referred to a text in the 'Further reading' section at the ends of these particular chapters. We have also included consumer and carer perspectives throughout the text in order to give emphasis to the importance of understanding the personal perspectives of the people we work with and for. This is partly in recognition of the changing role of consumers in health service delivery, but also in recognition of the increasing importance placed on consumer satisfaction and its link to quality of health care.

Currently, the two major diagnostic classification systems used in Australia and New Zealand, and internationally, are DSM-IV-TR (the *Diagnostic and Statistical Manual* of the American Psychiatric Association) and ICD-10-AM (the *International Classification of Diseases* from the World Health Organization). Although diagnostic labels can form a basis for shared understandings and more consistent management of mental health problems for health professionals as well as consumers/carers and families, they can also be restrictive and obscure the personal experiences and impacts of taking these medications. It is our intention, then, to maintain a balance between the science of psychotropics and the experience of taking and/or administering them.

The book is divided into three main sections:

Unit 1 (Ch 1–2) sets the context for the discussion by outlining the relevant clinical setting in which the medications are used in Australia and New Zealand, followed by an overview of the brain and how psychotropic medications work.

Unit 2 (Ch 3–6) provides an overview of each of the major groups of psychotropics and outlines their pathophysiology and pharmacology, identifies prescribing and administration issues for health professionals and discusses the perspectives of consumers and carers.

Unit 3 (Ch 7–8) is dedicated to addressing special issues, such as use of the psychotropic medications with people in special groups including pregnant and breastfeeding women and the elderly and the young, and also explores issues of relevance to the medications, such as use with agitated and aggressive people, adherence and administration issues like the use of PRN and depot preparations.

Kim Usher
Kim Foster
Shane Bullock

ABOUT THE AUTHORS

Professor Kim Usher, RN, RPN, DipNE, DipHSc, BA, MNSt, PhD, FCMHN, FRCNA, is Professor of Nursing at the Cairns campus of James Cook University, Queensland. Kim has considerable expertise in mental health nursing practice, education and research. She has had a passion for issues related to psychotropic medications since her time in clinical practice, which she further explored in her doctoral research. Kim has subsequently conducted numerous studies in the specialty area of psychotropic medication including issues related to PRN administration, use in pregnancy and breastfeeding and the metabolic syndrome. She has also published widely in this area and has two new PhD students about to embark on projects in the area of psychotropic medications. Kim has worked for the World Health Organization (WHO) as a consultant in the area of nursing on curriculum development and mental health and is currently a member of the Joint Asia Pacific Health Emergency Partners and Nursing Stakeholders Committee. She is also a member of many mental health nursing and related committees and working groups at both national and international levels. She has published widely in national and international journals, supervises a large number of PhD students and is an editor for *Collegian*, a Board Member of *Contemporary Nurse* and a reviewer for a number of high profile journals. In her spare time, Kim enjoys showing her German Shorthaired Pointer and Staffordshire Bull Terrier dogs with her partner.

Kim Foster, RN, RPN, DipAppSc(Nsg), BN, MA, PhD, FACMHN, MRCNA, is Associate Professor in the Faculty of Nursing and Midwifery at the University of Sydney, New South Wales. She has been involved in the education of nurses in the tertiary sector for 20 years, specialising in mental health nursing. Kim has also been a consultant to the WHO on psychosocial health education and to AusAID on mental health nursing education through the Fiji Health Sector Improvement Program. Her research interests include the perspectives of family/carers of people with mental illness; issues of the children of parents with mental illness; and the physical health of people with mental illness. Kim co-authored this book while Senior Lecturer in the School of Nursing, Midwifery and Nutrition at James Cook University, Cairns, Queensland and Associate Professor in the Faculty of Nursing and Midwifery at the University of Sydney, New

South Wales. Kim is also the co-author of a recent Australian textbook on mental health nursing for undergraduate nursing students.

Shane Bullock, BSc(Hons), PhD, is Associate Professor in the School of Veterinary and Biomedical Sciences at James Cook University, Townsville, Queensland. He has been involved in the education of health professionals for more than two decades. His expertise is within the neurosciences, more specifically neuropharmacology. His research interests include developing better treatments for Parkinson's disease, the phenomenon of brain lateralisation and the pharmacology knowledge of health professionals. Shane is a co-author of a successful textbook for students studying nursing and allied health professions called *Fundamentals of Pharmacology*, which is now in its fifth edition.

REVIEWERS

Stuart McLellan, RN Mental Health, Palliative Care Cert, Extended Care Cert
School of Nursing, Murdoch University, Western Australia

Jennifer Evans, RN, AssocDipArts (VocRehab), BHSc (Nursing), MNurSt, EdD
Lecturer, School of Nursing (NSW and ACT), Australian Catholic University

Stacey C Wilson, RN, MPhil, PGDipNsg (Mental Health)
Lecturer, School of Health and Social Services, Massey University, New Zealand

Meredith Bucknell, RN, RPN, BAppSci (Advanced Nursing), BEd, MNurs, FRCNA
Lecturer, School of Nursing, Deakin University

Michael Venning, PhD
Senior Lecturer, School of Pharmacy and Medical Sciences, University of South Australia

Rosemary Charleston, RPN, RN, BaHScNurs, MN, PhD Candidate
Lecturer, Centre for Psychiatric Nursing, School of Nursing and Social Work, University of Melbourne

Unit 1
Introduction and Background

CHAPTER 1

AN OVERVIEW OF PSYCHOPHARMACOLOGY

Objectives

The information in this chapter will assist you to:

» Understand the historical development of psychotropic medications and their impact on the treatment of mental disorders
» Identify the key periods when psychotropic medications were introduced
» Outline the clinical context in which psychotropic medications are used in Australia and New Zealand
» Understand the role of each health professional with regard to psychotropic medications
» Understand consumer and carer perspectives and experiences of taking psychotropic medications
» Describe the key ethical issues related to these medications

Key terms and abbreviations

24-hour crisis teams
Antipsychotic medication
Atypical antipsychotics
Consultancy teams
Continuing care
Deinstitutionalisation
First generation antipsychotics
Lithium
Mainstreaming
Psychiatric emergency services
Psychopharmacology

Psychotropic medications
Second generation antipsychotics
Typical antipsychotics
MAOIs – monoamine oxidase inhibitors
MITT – mobile intensive community treatment teams
NSRIs – noradrenaline serotonin reuptake inhibitors
SSRIs – selective serotonin reuptake inhibitors

PSYCHOPHARMACOLOGY – AN INTRODUCTION

The use of medications that affect thought processes and feeling states has been prevalent in the field of psychiatry for 60 years, since the introduction of lithium in 1949 by the Australian John Cade and the discovery of the efficacy of chlorpromazine in 1952. Commonly referred to as 'psychotropics', or medications affecting mood, perception and/or behaviour, these medications have elicited considerable controversy within the health sector and consumer groups while also bringing relief to consumers experiencing a range of often debilitating symptoms of mental health problems.

The following quote from a submission to the National Inquiry into the Human Rights of People with Mental Illness in Australia in 1993 (Healy & McNamara, in Burdekin et al 1993, p 238) expresses some of the tensions surrounding this group of medications:

> Psychotropic drugs have – and are intended to have – a significant impact on the way people think, feel and behave; that is, they are not only powerful and potentially therapeutic substances, but also intrusive and open to gross misuse … Their impact on personal and social functioning is typically severe … and, not infrequently, more disruptive to life than the original complaint.

Clearly, the introduction of lithium and then chlorpromazine, closely followed by other first generation antipsychotic medications, heralded a new era in psychiatry. This was referred to as the 'Golden Age' of psychopharmacology, rivalling the period of discovery, for instance, of antibiotics or antihypertensives (Lieberman et al 2000). There was, henceforth, a treatment for symptoms of psychosis that promised to give new hope to people who previously had had little relief from an almost continuous presence of symptoms and the related distressing emotions and behaviours they often brought. The introduction of medications that were able to control many of these symptoms contributed to a change in the care of people with mental illness, moving increasingly from large psychiatric institutions out into the community. In 1990, the ever-increasing focus on research and development in pharmacological treatments led to a declaration of the 'decade of the brain' (Floersch 2003). Neuroscience was becoming an ever more prominent force in understanding the structure and function of the brain, and how disturbances in neurochemical functioning could impact upon a person's thoughts, feelings and behaviours.

More recently, there have been further additions to the range of psychotropic medications. The second generation antipsychotics or atypicals were introduced initially in the 1950s and quickly withdrawn due to concerns over the side effects of clozapine. They were re-introduced in the 1980s and have brought with them comparable effectiveness to the first generation medications, yet with fewer side effects (Epstein et al 2007). This is a significant development, as the side effects of many of the psychotropics have been a major factor in consumer dissatisfaction and non-adherence. Similar developments occurred with the antidepressant group of medications. The tricyclic antidepressants and monoamine oxidase inhibitors (MAOIs) were introduced in the 1950s and were followed from the 1980s onwards by the newer and better tolerated selective serotonin reuptake inhibitors (SSRIs), for example fluoxetine, and the noradrenaline serotonin reuptake inhibitors (NSRIs), such as venlafaxine. However, concerns about the increasing costs of many of these medications and the social stigma and discrimination associated with the diagnosis and treatment of mental health problems, along with high side effect profiles, have contributed to consumers becoming increasingly vocal about perceived over-reliance on these forms of treatment. These concerns have existed within the context of a debate about the dominance of the scientific approach in the understanding and management of mental health problems.

The field of psychopharmacology is based on a model of understanding that considers that the development of symptoms of mental health problems is caused primarily by biochemical disturbances in the brain. The focus is on diagnosing the disorder/s in the individual, with the aim to cure or remediate symptoms through the use of somatic treatments such as psychotropic medications or electro-convulsive therapy. This has become the major paradigm in the care and treatment of people with mental health problems (Select Committee on Mental Health 2006). Yet, such an approach does not focus on the individual's experience of their illness and tends to emphasise their deficits rather than strengths. While biochemical causes are significant, there is an increasing understanding of the multifactorial influences of psychosocial factors on the development of mental health problems.

THE TREATMENT CONTEXT IN WHICH PSYCHOTROPIC MEDICATIONS ARE ADMINISTERED

As discussed, pharmacological treatments for mental disorders were extremely limited prior to the discoveries of the efficacies of psychotropic medications in the 1950s. As a consequence of these discoveries as well as changing sentiment regarding the treatment of mentally ill persons globally, reforms were implemented that led to a period where alternatives to institutionalisation for the care and treatment of people with severe mental illness were instigated. Known as 'deinstitutionalisation', this period led to the closure of most of the large psychiatric facilities in both Australia and New Zealand. In their place we now have mental health units attached to general hospitals, an approach referred to as 'mainstreaming', and a greater emphasis on community-based services.

As a direct result of deinstitutionalisation, the number of inpatient beds in public psychiatric facilities in Australia fell from around 30,000 in the 1960s to around 6,000 by 2005 (Department of Health and Ageing 2005). Inpatient services for people with severe mental illness in Australia and New Zealand are now mainly provided in general hospitals in intensive care, acute care and longer term care wards. Community services include psychiatric emergency services and 24-hour crisis teams, continuing care and consultancy teams and mobile intensive community treatment teams (MITT) and others (Muir-Cochrane et al 2005), although the terms used to describe the services may differ between areas, regions and countries. However, the investment in community mental health services promised at the time of deinstitutionalisation has not eventuated, resulting in a paucity of services for people experiencing a mental illness. In Australia, there continues to be an over-reliance on acute inpatient facilities as the primary, and sometimes only, source of support for people living with a serious mental illness and experiencing an acute episode (Mental Health Council of Australia 2006). This is a problem given that Australia and New Zealand both need more services for people requiring psychosis care. At present there are many such people who need to go to hospital but cannot because the acute units are full of people with chronic conditions (Andrews 2006).

Initiatives in Australia and New Zealand have been implemented in recent years in an attempt to improve the range of services available to people experiencing mental illness. In Australia, the National Mental Health Strategy launched a national reform agenda in recognition of the significant impact of mental illness on individuals, their families and the wider community. Under this strategy, the *National Mental Health Policy* (Australian Health Ministers 1992b) outlined the broad aims and goals designed to guide reform. The policy addressed important areas such as consumer rights, service mix, promotion and prevention. It also outlined the key principles underlying service developments, including the creation of opportunities for consumer participation in such developments and the need for responsiveness of the mental health services to the needs of consumers.

The *National Mental Health Plan* (Australian Health Ministers 1992a) set out a 5-year plan (1993–1998), which expressed commitment to the overarching principles of mainstreaming and integration. The *Second National Mental Health Plan* (1998–2003) and the *National Mental Health Plan* (2003–2008) have moved the reform agenda further, taking particular account of the range of settings in which health promotion and community education could occur, acknowledging that different people require different types of services and interventions, focusing on improving the quality and effectiveness of mental health services, supporting the development of partnerships between service providers and consumers and carers, increasing service responsiveness and fostering research, innovation and sustainability (Ash et al 2006). Regardless of the reform agenda, widespread dissatisfaction with mental health services in Australia continued and the Senate Select Committee was established in 2006. Its first report, *A National*

Approach to Mental Health; From Crisis to Community, outlined many issues such as the failure of deinstitutionalisation, recognition of the limitations of mainstreaming, the ineffective use of available resources, variability of the quality of mental health care, and how the dominant medical model continues to hinder improvement in the quality of services and care.

In New Zealand, deinstitutionalisation also led to recognition that community services were inadequate. As a result, the National Mental Health Strategy was launched in 1994 with the publication of *Looking Forward: Strategic Directions for the Mental Health Services* (Ministry of Health 1994). This publication outlined two goals: to decrease the prevalence of mental illness and mental health problems within the community; and to improve the health status of and reduce the impact of mental disorders on consumers, their families, caregivers and the general community. The directions of the strategy were to: implement community-based services; encourage Maori involvement in the planning, development and delivery of services; improve quality of care; balance personal rights with protection of the public; and develop a national drug and alcohol policy (Muir-Cochrane et al 2005). However, in 1996 the Mental Health Commission was established with the recognition that services had not achieved the desired outcomes and that a process of independent monitoring of mental health policy and service delivery was required to improve services. The Commission is guided by the 1998 document *Blueprint for Mental Health Services* and is charged with facilitating the implementation of the National Mental Health Strategy as well as reviewing aspects of services. The future direction for the delivery of mental health services in New Zealand is now guided by the *Te Tahuhu New Zealand Mental Health Plan* 2005–2015.

Within these treatment contexts, where there has been a push for the development and delivery of more services within the community, psychotropic medications have become increasingly important even though their use remains contentious (Frank et al 2005). However, disadvantaged social groups, such as Australian Indigenous peoples and New Zealand Maori and Pacific Islanders, are amongst those who have lower rates of access to mental health services and are therefore less likely to receive treatment, including psychotropic medication (O'Brien et al 2007, Wells et al 2006). The achievements of psychotropic medication research and development, however, have generally enabled people experiencing mental disorders to spend less time in hospital and to be troubled less by the deleterious side effects of the earlier psychotropic medications, making contemporary medicines much more acceptable to consumers (Epstein et al 2007).

LEGAL ISSUES WITH PSYCHOTROPIC MEDICATIONS

Being included in decision making about health care is considered a basic right, part of an individual's right to self-determination. It is important to remember that people with a mental illness have the same rights as everyone else when it comes to health care. In the past, the retention and treatment of a person involuntarily were passed off as a medical necessity. Today, however, lawyers are much more interested in the protection of the rights of the mentally ill and increasingly recognise how compulsory retention and treatment is a potential violation of a person's human and legal rights (Kerridge et al 2005). In Australia, each State and Territory has its own legislation designed to protect the rights of people with a mental disorder. This legislation (the Mental Health Acts) outlines the principles of treatment and care for people detained under the Act. Most Australian Mental Health Acts involve both voluntary and involuntary admission. In New Zealand, the appropriate legislation is the New Zealand Mental Health (Compulsory Assessment and Treatment) Act (1992), which provides the legal platform for current treatment within New Zealand.

When a consumer is admitted to an inpatient unit as an involuntary patient, this does not infer they should take no further part in decisions about their treatment. All patients have the right to be informed about decisions regarding their care and should be given the opportunity to participate in planning where appropriate. This right is just as important when the treatment is the administration of a psychotropic medication. It must also be realised that, even though a consumer's decision may at times be overruled by the treating team, this will not always be the case. Further, just because a person is deemed incompetent to make a particular decision, this does not imply they are incompetent of making any decision about their treatment (Kerridge et al 2005) – a consideration often overlooked by many health professionals. See Box 1.1 for human rights relating to psychotropic medications. For further information on the rights of people with mental illness with regard to their treatment, see the principles outlined by the United Nations for Human Rights on the website at the end of this chapter.

Greater emphasis on the consumer perspective in both Australia and New Zealand has seen the development of community-based treatment orders and other options that allow for the least restrictive option in the provision of appropriate care and treatment (Muir-Cochrane et al 2005). Community Treatment Orders are often used when a consumer responds well to psychotropic medication but is deemed highly likely to discontinue the medication when discharged. In such cases, the consumer may be placed under a Community Treatment Order so that they will be required

---

BOX 1.1 – HUMAN RIGHTS WITH REGARD TO PSYCHOTROPIC MEDICATIONS

Medication shall meet the best health needs of the patient, shall be given to a patient only for therapeutic or diagnostic purposes and shall never be administered as a punishment or for the convenience of others. Except for clinical trials, mental health practitioners shall only administer medication of known or demonstrated efficacy.

All medication shall be prescribed by a mental health practitioner authorised by law and shall be recorded in the patient's records.

(United Nations for Human Rights 1991; refer to United Nations for Human Rights website, http://www2.ohchr.org/english/law/principles.htm)

to attend a clinic for the administration of regular medication, thereby avoiding frequent re-admission. Over the past decade, consumers have increasingly shared their experiences of taking these medications and highlighted some of the major issues from their perspectives.

PERSPECTIVES ON PSYCHOTROPIC MEDICATIONS

CONSUMER/CARER PERSPECTIVES

Given the abundance of literature on the biomedical aspects of psychotropics, there has been a surprising lack of studies exploring consumer and/or carer perspectives on these medications. Yet, understanding the experiences of consumers and carers with psychotropics can inform the prescription and administration roles of health professionals, as well as enhancing their education and support of consumers and carers.

Consumers have reported on a number of aspects of taking psychotropics that can inform the practice of health professionals. These include the need to provide adequate information on side effects and the reasons for the medication, as well as telling consumers how long they will need to be on the medication (Happell et al 2004), as learning to live with the side effects is an integral aspect of the experience of taking them (Usher 2001). The role of health professionals in supporting consumers to manage their medications is also an important issue. The use of a non-hierarchical communication approach and attention to explaining possible side effects are two aspects of particular relevance (Happell et al 2004).

One consumer explains:

> I think it lessens the shock factor that happens when you start to get a side-effect if you know that you're – to expect them, you know, even things like dry mouth ... that affects how you see other people as well. Some medications your eyes are all back in the top of your head ... if you see that in someone else in the hospital and you don't know what it is, it can be very frightening and then you think ... if I take the medication will that happen to me?
>
> (Happell et al 2004, p 244)

In contrast, using a hierarchical approach to working with consumers has been related to issues of power, control and coercion in terms of prescribing, administering and taking these medications. Consumers have expressed concerns about feeling controlled by the medications themselves (Usher 2001) and about the external control that may be exerted by others such as family and friends. Consumers have perceived health professionals to be more focused on controlling the symptoms of their mental illness and enforcing their use of medication than on helping them to manage the side effects (Baker et al 2006, Happell et al 2004, Usher 2001). Conversely, though, consumers have reported feelings of personal control in terms of managing their symptoms if they have the opportunity to decide whether and how much medication they might need (Baker et al 2007). A consumer explains some of the reasons they take the medications:

> To try and stay on top of the situation and lead as much of a normal life as possible … to achieve what I want to achieve while I can and go where I want to in life.
>
> (Usher et al 2006)

The matter of who controls their use of medication is, however, also linked with consumers' non-adherence (or non-compliance) with psychotropics. Non-adherence remains a major issue in the administration and usage of these medications. There have been varying reports as to why consumers might not adhere to their prescribed medication regimens. These include difficulty accessing and paying for medications, that the side effects of the medications were problematic, that both taking the medications and having the side effects were embarrassing and stigmatising and deliberately making decisions not to take the medications because they did not need them or did not want to take them (Cooper et al 2007, Baker et al 2006, Muir-Cochrane et al 2006, Happell et al 2004). The issue of non-adherence will be explored further in later chapters. From a carer and family perspective, there is even less information on their views of psychotropic medications. Family members have reported being aware of consumers' concerns about their physical health, level of anxiety and discomfort while being on psychotropic medications. This has been linked with attendant issues such as quality of care and the help and support provided by health professionals (Hall-Lord et al 2003).

Table 1.1 outlines some of the benefits and disadvantages of psychotropic medications from a consumer perspective.

HEALTH PROFESSIONALS' ROLES AND PERSPECTIVES
Health professionals themselves have reported on their perceived roles and issues relating to the prescribing and administration of psychotropics

TABLE 1.1 – BENEFITS AND DISADVANTAGES OF PSYCHOTROPIC MEDICATIONS

Benefits	Disadvantages
Reduction or elimination of previously persistent psychotic, mood and/or behavioural symptoms	Side effects may be experienced by the consumer as more problematic than the original symptoms
Improvement in daily functioning as a result of reduction/elimination of symptoms, increased personal safety and reduction in potential risk to others	Poorer quality of life because of reduced ability to perform daily functions due to side effects such as sedation, etc.
Reduced stigma and discrimination due to absence of symptoms	Increased stigma and discrimination due to having to take psychotropic medications and due to their side effects
Improved quality of life and sense of wellbeing due to reduction/removal of symptoms; enhanced self-esteem	Access to, and paying the costs of, the medications can be difficult
Greater feeling of self-control and self-efficacy due to the decision to take the medications	Feeling controlled and/or coerced by others to take medications in order to manage the symptoms of the mental health problem

THINKING CHALLENGE 1.1

Consider the medications from the perspective of taking them yourself. What might it be like to have to take a number of oral medications daily and/or receive regular injections? What would it be like to experience drowsiness on a daily basis or weight gain due to the medication? How might these and other issues affect your attitude towards taking psychotropics?

In terms of control over the usage of psychotropics – how can health professionals balance the consumer's right to decide what treatments they receive with their responsibility to provide safe and effective care?

and the monitoring and evaluation of psychotropic medication use.

In terms of psychotropic medications, key health professionals and their roles include:

- **Medical officers, general practitioners and psychiatrists** Doctors have a primary role in the prescription of psychotropics for consumers and monitoring their use in general health settings, as well as in specialist mental health settings, in public and private facilities, and in inpatient and community settings.
- **Nurses, particularly mental health nurses and mental health nurse practitioners** Nurses working in all health care settings are likely to work with consumers taking psychotropic medications;

however, mental health nurses and mental health nurse practitioners have a primary role in assessment, administration of medication, monitoring of effects and managing problems and difficulties with taking psychotropics. Nurse practitioners have further specialist roles including prescribing a certain range of medications, ordering of diagnostic tests and referral to specialists.

- **Midwives and maternal child health nurses** Midwives and maternal child health nurses work with pregnant, labouring and breastfeeding women and their families in both hospital and community settings and are often working with women who are taking, or will be prescribed, psychotropic medications. They therefore need a good understanding of the effects, potential interactions, side effects and potential effects on the baby if the mother is taking psychotropic medications.
- **Pharmacists** Pharmacists have a primary role in the storage, supply and distribution of medication in hospital or retail pharmacies. They are responsible for ensuring that medications are safely stored and dispensed according to the law and for providing consumers with information about their medications, checking for potential drug interactions or misuse and advising consumers about safe storage and usage.
- **Psychologists** Although psychologists are not authorised to prescribe or administer medication, they often work with consumers who are taking psychotropics and therefore need to have a good understanding of the effects and side effects of the medications in order to work most effectively with their clients.
- **Social workers** Social workers focus on issues relating to social justice and work in a range of mental health and other services alongside other members of the multidisciplinary team, performing roles such as case management, counselling and therapy. Similarly to psychologists, while they are not authorised to prescribe or administer psychotropic medications, their work with mental health consumers necessitates a good understanding of the medications.
- **Occupational therapists** Occupational therapists work with consumers who have a range of psychosocial issues and assist them to carry out activities of daily living, including driving, cooking and so on, and also provide specific therapies such as diversion therapy. Although they are not authorised to administer or monitor psychotropic medications, their work with consumers requires them to have a thorough understanding of the effects, potential interactions and side effects of these medications.
- **Health workers** There are different levels of preparation for health

workers in the mental health system but, generally, health workers perform roles that include liaising with families, detecting issues with medications, providing advocacy for (and a link between) other health professionals and Indigenous consumers and families, and ensuring that education on social and emotional health issues is understood by consumers, families and their communities.

From a health professional's perspective, the issues relating to prescribing, administering and monitoring psychotropic medications share some similarities with those expressed by consumers, but also a number of differences. Clearly, health professionals – particularly doctors and nurses – can be informed by consumers' experiences, as some of their understandings of the benefits of psychotropic medications are not matched by consumers'.

Some doctors, for instance, have reported that, while they consider the risks associated with particular medications, their effectiveness in assisting consumers to remain functional makes them a less problematic solution than other options. Doctors have also reported they do not often see the side effects of the medications, and that consumers often do not report them, so doctors' perceptions of positive risk–benefit ratios are reinforced. Some doctors have reported their skepticism towards non-pharmacological approaches to symptoms of mental illness, such as anxiety, and stated that they consider psychotropics to be the most effective way to help the person (Damestoy et al 1999).

Mental health nurses, on the other hand, have reported that they understand that part of their role and responsibilities is to educate and support consumers taking psychotropics and their families (Happell et al 2002, Allen 1998), but that they sometimes assume consumers have good knowledge of the medications. Nurses have often had to self-educate themselves on the medications due to a lack of available in-service education, and have experienced barriers to performing their roles with respect to psychotropics due to factors such as high client turnover, lack of a structured approach to care plans and high doctor turnover (Happell et al 2002).

Some differences have been found between the views of doctors and nurses on psychotropic medications. These include differences in views on which symptoms or behaviours may indicate the need for medication, with nurses being more likely, for example, to consider psychotic symptoms such as delusions and hallucinations as indicative of the need to administer psychotropics. However, both doctors and nurses have been found to have some incorrect beliefs concerning the uses for particular psychotropics and have shown some reluctance, for instance, to use benzodiazepines for acute psychotic symptoms, even though these have been found to be effective (Geffen et al 2002).

However, our view on the role of health professionals is that we all work together in multidisciplinary settings where collaboration is important and offers the best potential outcomes for consumers. It is the responsibility of each health professional to be cognisant of developments in psychotropic medications, to understand drug actions and possible side effects and to apply this knowledge to their work with consumers. All health professionals need to be respectful of consumers' and carers' perspectives and experiences with psychotropic medications, and to take their complaints and concerns seriously. Given the growing role of consumer satisfaction in determining quality health care, including consumers and respecting their views on all facets of treatment is essential for all health professionals.

CONCLUSIONS

This chapter has provided the reader with an overview of the historical development of psychotropic medication and outlined the current context in which these medications are used within Australia and New Zealand, including the roles of health professionals involved in their administration. The chapter also offered a short synopsis of the relevant ethical issues related to the prescription and administration of psychotropic medications. Finally, the important role of consumers and carers was outlined. The remainder of the book is outlined below.

Chapter 2: Overview of the brain and pharmacological principles. In this chapter the overall brain structures and functions relating to mental state and behaviour are explained, and the mechanisms and principles by which psychotropic medications act are described.

Chapters 3 to 6 provide a holistic overview that includes: why and how the medications work, contemporary information on the latest medications being used plus information on older types of medication where appropriate; an overview of the side effects and their management; and issues related to administration such as adherence, clinical issues and interactions. Case studies will be used throughout these chapters to assist the reader's understanding of the issues related to each medication.

Chapter 3: Medications used for disturbances in cognition and perception. The chapter identifies the clinical features of common disturbances in cognition and perception, describes the pharmacology of medications used to treat these symptoms, and outlines prescribing and administration issues.

Chapter 4: Medications used for disturbances in mood and affect. The chapter identifies the clinical features of common disturbances in mood and affect, describes the pharmacology of medications used to treat these symptoms and outlines prescribing and administration issues.

Chapter 5: Medications used for anxiety and sleep disturbances. The chapter identifies the clinical features of common disturbances in anxiety and sleep, describes the pharmacology of medications used to treat these symptoms and outlines prescribing and administration issues.

Chapter 6: Medications used for substance misuse. The chapter identifies the clinical features of common substance use issues, describes the pharmacology of medications used to treat these symptoms and outlines prescribing and administration issues.

Chapter 7: Issues related to the prescription and use of psychotropic medication in special populations. Psychotropic use in special populations is discussed, including psychotropic drug use in older persons, pregnant and/or breastfeeding women, children and young people, and the Indigenous peoples of Australia and New Zealand. Ethical issues as they relate to each group are also discussed.

Chapter 8: Special issues with the use of psychotropic medications. Issues discussed include the management of behavioural emergencies such as violent and aggressive behaviours, the use of PRN and depot psychotropic medications, the management of serious medication side effects such as metabolic syndrome, the experience and management of sexual dysfunction related to psychotropic medications and the issue of polypharmacy.

Useful websites

New Zealand Mental Health Commission – providing information on the New Zealand treatment context, http://www.mhc.org.nz

The New Zealand Mental Health Foundation – providing information on mental health consumer groups, http://www.mhf.org.nz

United Nations for Human Rights – containing 'Principles for the protection of persons with mental illness and the improvement of mental health care' document, http://www2.ohchr.org/english/law/principles.htm

Recommended reading

Ash D, Brown P, Burvill P et al 2007 Mental Health Services in Australia. In: Meadows G, Singh B, Grigg M (eds) Mental Health in Australia, Collaborative Community Practice, 2nd edn. Oxford University Press, Melbourne, pp 99–131

Happell B, Manias E, Roper C 2004 Wanting to be heard: mental health consumers' experiences of information about medication. International Journal of Mental Health Nursing 13(4):242–248

Muir-Cochrane E, O'Brien A, Wand T 2005 The Australian and New Zealand

Politico-Legal Context. In: Elder R, Evans K, Nizette D (eds) Psychiatric and
Mental Health Nursing. Elsevier, Sydney, pp 45–61
O'Brien A P, Boddy J, Hardy D J 2007 Culturally specific process measures to
improve mental health clinical practice: Indigenous focus. Australia and New
Zealand Journal of Psychiatry 41:667–674

Teaching and learning activities

* Most professionals who work in the area of psychiatry would say that the
introduction of psychotropic medications has revolutionised the treatment
of mental disorders. However, due to the adverse effects and other issues
related to taking these medications, consumers may have different ideas. Try to
imagine what it would be like for a consumer who expresses a desire not to take
psychotropic medications when faced with clinicians who believe they are the
answer to mental disorder.
* Ethical issues related to the administration of psychotropic medications are often
issues of autonomy or choice. Can you identify the main concerns that consumers
might express regarding these issues?

References

Allen J 1998 A survey of psychiatric nurses' opinions of advanced practice roles in
psychiatric nursing. Journal of Psychiatric and Mental Health Nursing
5(6):451–462
Andrews G 2006 Implications for intervention and prevention from the New
Zealand and Australian mental health surveys. Australian and New Zealand
Journal of Psychiatry 40:827–829
Ash D, Benson A, Dunbar L et al 2006 Mental Health Services in Australia. In:
Meadows G, Singh B, Grigg M (eds) Mental Health in Australia, Collaborative
Community Practice, 2nd edn. Oxford University Press, Melbourne, pp 63–98
Australian Health Ministers 1992a The National Mental Health Plan. Australian
Government Publishing Service, Canberra
Australian Health Ministers 1992b National Mental Health Policy. Australian
Government Publishing Service, Canberra
Baker J, Lovell K, Easton K et al 2006 Service users' experiences of 'as needed'
psychotropic medications in acute mental healthcare settings. Journal of
Advanced Nursing 56(4):354–362
Baker J, Lovell K, Harris N et al 2007 Multidisciplinary consensus of best practice for
pro re nata (PRN) psychotropic medications within acute health settings: a Delphi
study. Journal of Psychiatric and Mental Health Nursing 14:478–484
Burdekin B, Guilfoyle M, Hall D 1993 Human Rights and Equal Opportunities
Commission. Human rights and mental illness: Report of the National Inquiry
into the Human Rights of People with Mental Illness (vol 1). Australian
Government Publishing Service, Canberra

Cooper C, Bebbington P, King M et al 2007 Why people do not take their psychotropic drugs as prescribed: Results of the 2000 National Psychiatric Morbidity Survey. Acta Psychiatrica Scandinavica 1(7) (OnlineEarly articles) doi:10.1111/j.1600-0447.2006.00974.x

Damestoy N, Collin J, Lalande R 1999. Prescribing psychotropic medication for elderly patients: some physicians' perspectives. Canadian Medical Association Journal 161(2):143–145

Department of Health and Ageing 2005 National Mental Health Report 2005: Summary of Ten Years of Reform in Australia's Mental Health Services under the National Mental Health Strategy 1993-2003 (Ninth Report). Commonwealth of Australia, Canberra

Epstein M, McDermott F, Meadows G et al 2007 Society, mental health, and illness. In: Meadows G, Singh B, Grigg M (eds) Mental Health in Australia: Collaborative Community Practice, Oxford University Press, Melbourne, pp 3–11

Floersch J 2003 The subjective experience of youth psychotropic treatment. Social Work in Mental Health 1(4):51–69

Frank R G, Conti R M, Goldman H H 2005 Mental Health Policy and Psychotropic Drugs. The Milbank Quarterly 83(2):271–298

Geffen J, Cameron A, Sorenson L et al 2002 Pro re nata medication for psychoses: the knowledge and beliefs of doctors and nurses. Australian and New Zealand Journal of Psychiatry 36(5):642–648

Hall-Lord M L, Johansson I, Schmidt I et al 2003 Family members' perceptions of pain and distress related to analgesics and psychotropic drugs, and quality of care for elderly nursing home residents. Health and Social Care in the Community 11(3):262–274

Happell B, Manias E, Pinikahana J 2002 The role of the inpatient mental health nurse in facilitating patient adherence to medication regimes. International Journal of Mental Health Nursing 11(4):251–259

Happell B, Manias E, Roper C 2004 Wanting to be heard: mental health consumers' experiences of information about medication. International Journal of Mental Health Nursing 13(4):242–248

Kerridge I, Lowe M, McPhee J 2005 Ethics and Law for the Health Professions, 2nd edn. The Federation Press, Leichhardt, NSW

Lieberman J A, Golden R, Stroup S et al 2000 Drugs of the psychopharmacological revolution in clinical psychiatry. Psychiatric Services 51(10):1254–1258

Mental Health Council of Australia 2006 Smart Services: Innovative Models of Mental Health Care in Australia and New Zealand. Mental Health Council of Australia

Ministry of Health 1994 Looking Forward: Strategic Directions for the Mental Health Services. Ministry of Health, Wellington, New Zealand

Muir-Cochrane E, O'Brien A, Wand T 2005 The Australian and New Zealand Politico-Legal Context. In: Elder R, Evans K, Nizette D (eds) Psychiatric and

Mental Health Nursing. Elsevier, Sydney, pp 45–61

Muir-Cochrane E, Fereday J, Jureidini J et al 2006 Self-management of medication for mental health problems by homeless young people. International Journal of Mental Health Nursing 15(3):163–170

O'Brien A P, Boddy J, Hardy D J 2007 Culturally specific process measures to improve mental health clinical practice: Indigenous focus. Australia and New Zealand Journal of Psychiatry 41:667–674

Select Committee on Mental Health 2006 Senate Committee Report: A national approach to mental health – from crisis to community. Senate Printing Unit, Parliament House, Canberra

Usher K 2001 Taking neuroleptic medications as the treatment for schizophrenia: A phenomenological study. Australian and New Zealand Journal of Mental Health Nursing 10(3):145–155

Usher K, Hay P, Quirk F et al 2006 Development of a questionnaire to measure antipsychotic medication compliance. Paper presented at the 32nd International Conference of the Australian and New Zealand College of Mental Health Nurses, Alice Springs, October

Wells J E, Oakley Browne M A, Scott K M et al 2006 Te Rau Hinengaro: The New Zealand Mental Health Survey: overview of methods and findings. Australia and New Zealand Journal of Psychiatry 40:835–844

CHAPTER 2

AN OVERVIEW OF THE BRAIN AND PHARMACOLOGICAL PRINCIPLES

Objectives

The information in this chapter will assist you to:

» Name the four principal parts of the human brain and the important regions within each part
» Briefly outline the major functions of the principal parts of the brain
» Identify the structural and functional unit of the brain and outline the nature of its connections
» Describe the process of neurotransmission and outline the roles of the major brain transmitters
» Name the major cellular processes targeted by psychotropic agents in general
» State the factors that influence drug absorption and the distribution of drugs across the blood–brain barrier
» Indicate how plasma protein binding influences drug action
» Outline the role of cytochrome P450 enzymes and the consequences of liver/renal impairment on psychotropic drug effects
» Describe how hepatic first-pass effects influence oral administered drugs
» Appreciate how genetic make-up and ethnicity can influence drug pharmacokinetics

Key terms and abbreviations

Brain stem
Cerebellum
Cerebrum
Diencephalon
Neurone
Neurotransmitter
Pharmacodynamics
Pharmacogenetics

Pharmacokinetics
5-HT – 5-hydroxytryptamine
ACh – acetylcholine
BBB – blood–brain barrier
CNS – central nervous system
CYP – cytochrome P450 enzymes
GABA – gamma-aminobutyric acid

INTRODUCTION

In order to understand how psychotropic drugs bring about changes in affect, perception, cognition and/or behaviour an introduction to the way in which the brain is organised and processes information is required. The information in this chapter will provide a reference point for the discussions of pathophysiological processes and the properties of important drug groups that follow in later chapters.

The human brain is a most extraordinary structure. More than any other body organ, it represents the essence of our humanness and distinguishes us from the rest of the animal kingdom. It can be simply yet elegantly described as our body's organ of thought. However, this phrase greatly understates its purpose in our lives. In addition to regulating body function, the brain is the seat of the intellect. Among its diverse functions it solves problems, allows communication, constructs our personality and temperament, generates emotions and behaviour, affords us a conscious awareness of sensations, initiates voluntary movement, stores memories and provides a sense of self.

An adult human brain is not unlike a giant-sized walnut in appearance, weighing approximately a kilogram with a consistency similar to that of jelly and the colouring of strawberry yoghurt. The tissues of the brain are easily damaged. It is interesting that the most fascinating and complex of human organs, holding a lifetime of thoughts and experiences, turns out to be so fragile and insubstantial.

ORGANISATION OF THE BRAIN

The four principal parts of the brain are the cerebrum, diencephalon, brain stem and cerebellum (see Fig 2.1).

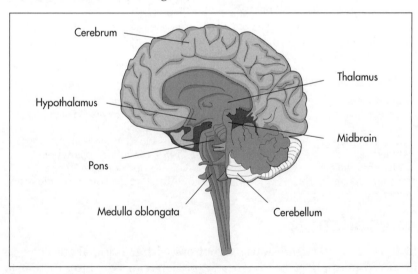

Figure 2.1 – The principal parts of the brain.
A sagittal cross-section indicating the principal parts located within the right side of the human brain.
Adapted from Fundamentals of Pharmacology (5th edn), 2007, by S Bullock, E Manias and A Galbraith, Prentice Hall, Fig 33.1, p 351, with permission

CEREBRUM

The cerebrum is the largest part of the human brain and its surface is rippled with shallow grooves and ridges that afford the characteristic walnut-like appearance – these undulations increase the surface area of the cerebrum to provide greater processing power. The surface crust of the cerebrum is about 3 mm thick and is called the cerebral cortex. A deep midline groove separates the cerebrum into equal halves called cerebral hemispheres. Communication between hemispheres is achieved via a number of commissures or connecting bridges of nerve fibres, the biggest of these being the corpus callosum. The hemispheres can be further subdivided into lobes, of which there are four external and one internal. The four external are called the frontal, parietal, temporal and occipital lobes; the internal one, tucked in deep between the frontal and temporal lobes, is called the insula (see Fig 2.2).

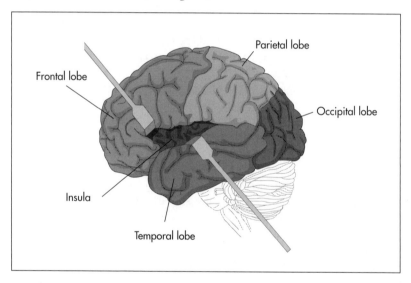

Figure 2.2 – Lobes of the human brain.
Adapted from Human Anatomy and Physiology (7th edn), 2007, by E N Marieb and K Hoehn, Pearson-Benjamin Cummings, Fig 12.6, p 435, with permission

The cerebral cortex is organised in such a way as to allow specialisation of function. Discrete regions of the cortex control the primary processing of vision, taste, hearing, general sensations and muscle movements. Furthermore, as new information is received it can be referenced against past experiences stored in association areas. The frontal lobes are particularly important in the processing of emotions and behaviour, decision making, personality and temperament, self-discipline and cognition. Another form of specialisation occurs at the hemispheric level: one hemisphere may be more dominant over the other in the control of some functions. Classic examples of this cerebral dominance include handedness (90% of humans are right-handed), language control (left hemisphere is usually dominant) and spatial perception (right hemisphere is usually dominant). This phenomenon does not mean that the non-dominant hemisphere makes no contribution to these functions, nor does it mean that in a typical right-handed person their left hemisphere is dominant for all of these functions – it is very much function-specific. In some brain disorders, such as schizophrenia and depression, an imbalance between the hemispheres may contribute to the manifestation of the condition (see Chs 3 and 4).

DIENCEPHALON

The diencephalon contains the thalamus and hypothalamus. The thalamus is a relay centre for both ascending (sensory) and descending (motor) information. Sensations from the body enter the thalamus and are sorted as to the origin of the transmission and the type of sensation received (e.g., taste, touch, vibration or thermal). They can then be sent to the appropriate processing centre in the cortex, where sensory perception is completed. The hypothalamus has a significant role to play in homeostasis with respect to appetite regulation, fluid and electrolyte balance and body temperature control. It is the interface between the nervous and the endocrine systems, in that it is physically connected to the pituitary gland by a stalk and has a great influence on hormone release from this gland. The hypothalamus also plays a role in autonomic nervous system control. The link between the hypothalamus and the autonomic nervous system, pituitary gland and other brain regions affords it a unique role in the initiation of emotional and behavioural responses.

BRAIN STEM AND CEREBELLUM

The brain stem consists of three regions: midbrain, pons and medulla. It is associated with the control of a number of important reflexes (e.g. head movements, tracking stimuli, vision, coughing and vomiting), as well as vital functions such as respiration, blood pressure and heart rate. The major motor pathway serving the skeletal muscles passes through the posterior portion of the medulla. This region is called the medullary pyramids because of the characteristic appearance of the posterior surface of the medulla. Another name for this motor tract is the pyramidal pathway.

The cerebellum has a major role in muscle movement. It assists in the planning of movements, provides feedback to the cortex as to the efficiency of the initiated movements, is involved in the control of posture and muscle tone and ensures that movements are smooth and coordinated.

NEURONAL COMMUNICATION

NERVE CELLS AND PATHWAYS

Communication around the nervous system occurs via the activation of nerve pathways. The structural and functional unit of these pathways is the neurone or nerve cell. There are billions of neurones in the human brain. Neurones receive messages from other nerve cells in the form of electrical impulses and respond by either sending or not sending impulses along to the next neurone in the pathway. Neurone function is also influenced by chemical modulators within the tissue fluid bathing the nerve cells. Circuits of nerve pathways connect regions of the brain; many circuits form nerve networks that control brain functions. Brain circuits and networks can be switched on or off as they process inputs, integrate information, make decisions and activate the most appropriate responses. Thought processes and life experiences can reinforce and enhance the dominance of particular brain circuits at the cost of others. Indeed, our brains are quite malleable. Throughout our lives, neural connections are changing; new connections between neurones are made and connections in existing circuits are lost. This is the basis of learning and memory formation. It is a requirement in the normal development and maturation of humans to adulthood, but this process continues throughout adult life as we learn to adapt to changing life circumstances.

NEUROTRANSMISSION

The interface or connection between sending and receiving neurones is called the synapse. It has been suggested that there are 1×10^{15} synapses in the human brain. The synapse consists of the axon terminal of the sending neurone (the presynaptic neurone), the cell membrane of the receiving neurone (the postsynaptic neurone) and a small gap between the two called the synaptic cleft (see Fig 2.3). As the presynaptic and postsynaptic neurones do not actually make direct contact, the communication is conveyed postsynaptically via the release of chemical messengers or neurotransmitters.

The manner in which one neurone communicates with the next neurone in the pathway is called neurotransmission. The main phases of neurotransmission are the release of neurotransmitter from the presynaptic axon terminal, interaction of the transmitter with postsynaptic receptors and inactivation of the neurotransmitter. There are two main ways in which neurotransmitters can be inactivated. An enzyme may be present in the synaptic cleft that breaks down the transmitter once it has been released from the axon terminal. Alternatively, the released transmitter can be removed from the synaptic

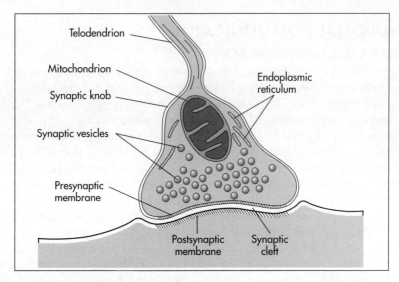

Figure 2.3 – The synapse.
A representation of a typical synapse.
Reproduced from Fundamentals of Anatomy and Physiology *(7th edn), 2006, by
F H Martini, Pearson Education, Inc (publishing as Benjamin Cummings), Fig 12.2,
with permission*

cleft via a re-uptake pump embedded in the membrane of the axon
terminal or surrounding supporting cells.

NEUROTRANSMITTERS

The most abundant neurotransmitters in the central nervous system are
glutamate and gamma-aminobutyric acid (GABA). Glutamate is excitatory,
in that it triggers depolarisation of the postsynaptic neurone resulting in
impulse conduction, whereas GABA is inhibitory in that it hyperpolarises
the postsynaptic membrane and inhibits impulse conduction along the
pathway.

Other important brain neurotransmitters include: acetylcholine, which
has a role in cognition and memory; noradrenaline, which is involved
in arousal, mood and sleep; dopamine, which is involved in the control
of behaviour, emotions, hormone release and motor function; and
serotonin (5-hydroxytryptamine or 5-HT), which has roles in arousal,
mood, behaviour and pain perception. In some areas of the brain these
transmitters act to increase activity in nerve circuits, in others they inhibit
the circuit. This action, either circuit inhibition or activation, is determined
by the subtype of the neurotransmitter receptor that is present. For all of
the neurotransmitters mentioned above, at least two subtypes of receptor
have been identified. A summary of the major neurotransmitters and their

receptor subtypes is provided in Table 2.1. In later chapters you will see that a number of common mental health illnesses have been linked to neurotransmitter imbalances.

TABLE 2.1 - MAJOR NEUROTRANSMITTERS AND THEIR RECEPTOR SUB-TYPES		
Neurotransmitter	**Receptor sub-types**	**Brain functions**
Acetylcholine (ACh)	Nicotinic Muscarinic ($M_1 - M_5$)	Motor control, cognition, memory
Noradrenaline (NA)	Alpha (α_1, α_2) Beta ($\beta_1, \beta_2, \beta_3$)	Affect, consciousness, appetite, body temperature control
Dopamine (DA)	$D_1 - D_5$	Motor control, vomiting, pituitary hormone release, behaviour
Serotonin (5-HT)	$5\text{-HT}_1 - 5\text{-HT}_7$	Consciousness, affect, behaviour, pain modulation
Glutamate	N-methyl-D-aspartate (NMDA) Kainate α-Amino-3-hydroxy-5-methyl-isoxazole (AMPA)	Learning, memory
Gamma-aminobutyric acid (GABA)	$GABA_A$ $GABA_B$	Consciousness, motor control, memory, learning

PRINCIPLES OF PHARMACOLOGICAL ACTION WITH RESPECT TO PSYCHOTROPIC DRUGS

We will deal with the specific mechanisms of action of important psychotropic drug groups in relation to the disorders for which they are used as treatments in later chapters. Here, we present some general pharmacodynamic principles.

PHARMACODYNAMICS

Drugs produce their action on the nervous system by targeting certain cellular processes involved in impulse generation and conduction, and/or neurotransmission. Generally, the major psychotropic agents that you encounter in clinical practice are believed to act by altering the activities of receptors, enzymes, ion channels and chemical transporter systems involved in these processes (see Fig 2.4). In order to approximate normal brain functioning some drugs activate these targets, while others inhibit them.

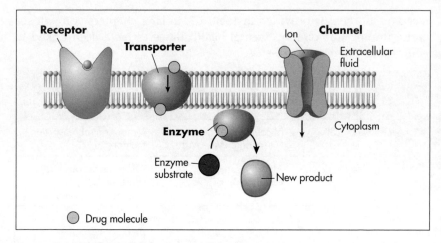

Figure 2.4 – Common cellular targets of drug action.
Drug molecules can bind to these cellular targets to either facilitate or inhibit the normal response in order to bring about the desired clinical effect.
Adapted from Neuroscience: Exploring the Brain (3rd edn), 2007, by M F Bear, B W Connors and M A Paradiso, Lippincott, Williams and Watkins, Fig 5.16, p 119, with permission

Interestingly, there is growing evidence that some established psychotropic agents may also alter the availability of nerve growth factors and that their beneficial actions may be explained, at least in part, by an alteration in neuronal connectivity (see Ch 4).

PHARMACOKINETICS

When a drug is administered to a person it is subjected to a number of physiological processes as it passes through the body. The study of these processes is called pharmacokinetics and involves the phases of drug absorption, distribution, metabolism and elimination. Here is a brief overview of pharmacokinetics and its implications for clinical management of drug therapy.

Drug absorption

The drug absorption phase is characterised by the transfer of a drug into the bloodstream via its route of administration. Examples of this are the movement from gut to blood after oral drug administration or the movement from hypodermis to blood after subcutaneous drug injection. The rate of absorption may vary for different routes of administration and this depends on the accessibility of the site of administration to the bloodstream and the rate of blood flow. Factors affecting drug absorption generally include drug solubility (lipid solubility enhances absorption because cell membranes are predominantly composed of lipids), molecular size (small molecules are more easily absorbed), blood flow and the presence of cellular transporter systems. Solubility may be influenced by the pH of the body compartment that the drug has entered. The drug molecules may be predominantly charged or uncharged, depending on the pH of the compartment. Generally speaking, a drug that is a weak acid will be predominantly uncharged (and relatively more lipid soluble) in an acidic environment and charged (less soluble) in an alkaline (or basic) environment. A drug that is a weak base will be more lipid soluble in an alkaline environment (see Fig 2.5).

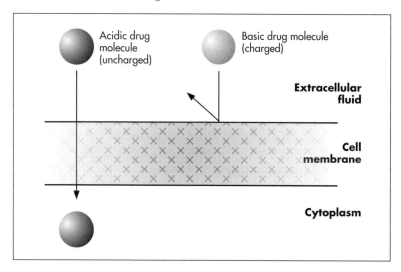

Figure 2.5 – The effects of pH on drug solubility.
The pH of the body compartment influences the proportion of drug molecules that are either charged or uncharged. A charged particle has difficulty crossing into an adjacent body compartment, whereas an uncharged particle has greater lipid solubility. Generally, an acidic drug in an acidic environment has a greater proportion of uncharged particles and can cross a membrane more easily than a basic drug.

Important factors influencing drug absorption from the gastrointestinal tract include the degree of gastrointestinal motility (slower motility allows more time for drug absorption), the rate of gastric emptying (a faster rate places the drug in the small intestines more quickly, which is the site where most absorption occurs), as well as the presence of food or other chemicals in the gastrointestinal tract that might impede absorption. Most drug absorption occurs in the small intestine because of the large surface area of this region.

Drug distribution

Once in the bloodstream psychotropic drugs must be able to cross into the central nervous system (CNS) in order to interact with the appropriate drug target. The structural organisation of the blood capillaries supplying the brain is different from that in other body regions, establishing a physical barrier to drug absorption. This blood–brain barrier (BBB) excludes many drugs from entering the CNS. There are other natural physiological barriers to drug entry including the placenta and testes. The use of psychotropic drugs during pregnancy and breastfeeding is dealt with in Chapter 7. Generally speaking, greater lipid solubility, small molecular size and/or the presence of cellular transporter systems for that drug afford better penetration through the BBB.

Plasma protein binding

Drugs with relatively poor solubility in blood (lipid soluble drugs and weak acids) may be able to bind to plasma proteins and so be more easily transported around the body. The most important plasma protein for this purpose is albumin. Protein binding is expressed as a percentage of the total drug present in the bloodstream. When the percentage of drug binding is greater than 60%, it is considered strongly bound. While bound to plasma protein the drug cannot induce its action nor can it be broken down. Only the free drug in the blood can exert its pharmacological effect. The proportions of free and bound drug remain in equilibrium (see Fig 2.6). Thus, plasma proteins act as drug reservoirs, prolonging the duration of action of the drug in the body. When two drugs that bind strongly to plasma proteins are present in the body at the same time, they may compete against each other for the limited number of protein binding sites. The consequence is that there will be more free drug molecules in the blood exerting a stronger, possibly toxic, pharmacological effect than expected. The dose of one or both drugs may have to be adjusted. Examples of psychotropic drugs that bind strongly to plasma proteins are provided in Table 2.2.

Drug metabolism

The main site of drug metabolism is the liver. Drugs are metabolised to make them more water-soluble in urine so that they can be eliminated. Metabolic processes are completed primarily through the action of enzymes, where the chemical structure of a drug is altered by removing parts of the molecule or adding new parts to it. Another means of drug metabolism is to join an inert substance to the drug molecule; this is called conjugation. Altering a drug's molecular structure usually results in changes in its pharmacological activity.

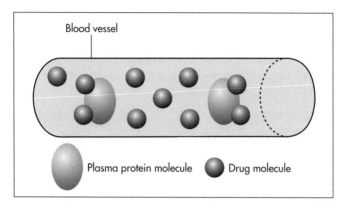

Figure 2.6 – Simplified representation of plasma protein binding.
Drug binding to plasma proteins is represented in this diagram. The proportion of bound drug molecules is in equilibrium with free molecules. In this example, the drug is 40% protein-bound.
Reproduced from Fundamentals of Pharmacology (5th edn), 2007, by S Bullock, E Manias and A Galbraith, Prentice Hall, Fig 14.4, p 142, with permission

TABLE 2.2 – EXAMPLES OF PSYCHOTROPIC DRUGS THAT BIND STRONGLY TO PLASMA PROTEINS	
Psychotropic drug group	Examples
Tricyclic antidepressants	Imipramine, amitryptyline, doxepin
First generation antipsychotic agents	Chlorpromazine, thioridazine
Antianxiety (anxiolytic) agents and hypnotics	Oxazepam, diazepam, temazepam
Antidepressants called selective serotonin reuptake inhibitors (SSRIs)	Fluoxetine, paroxetine, citalopram

CYTOCHROME P450 ENZYMES

An important set of enzymes involved in drug metabolism is the cytochrome P450 (CYP) family, which is predominately located in the liver. A small number of CYP enzymes are involved in the metabolism of hundreds of medicines, including many important psychotropic agents. Interestingly, the presence of particular drugs in the body can alter the activity of a CYP enzyme involved in the metabolism of other drugs. Such drug interactions can have a significant effect on the duration and magnitude of action of an administered medicine. These interactions can result in poor metabolism of a CYP-dependent drug, leading to increased and prolonged drug effects, or induce an interaction of a different kind where more rapid metabolism results in lower than expected and shorter lived drug effects. For the psychotropic agents important drug interactions are associated with the induction or inhibition of certain subgroupings of CYP enzymes, including CYPD2, CYPD19 and CYPA1 isoforms. Examples of important psychotropic drug interactions associated with CYP enzyme metabolism are provided in Table 2.3.

TABLE 2.3 – EXAMPLES OF CYP-BASED PSYCHOTROPIC DRUG INTERACTIONS		
CYP-dependent drug	Drugs that induce CYP metabolism of these drugs	Drugs that inhibit CYP metabolism of these drugs
Second generation antipsychotic agents (clozapine, olanzapine) Tricyclic antidepressants (amitryptyline, imipramine)	Tobacco smoking Anticonvulsant agents (phenytoin, carbamazepine)	Antimicrobial agents (ciprofloxacin, erythromycin)
Selective serotonin reuptake inhibitor (SSRI) (fluoxetine)	Anticonvulsant agents (phenytoin, carbamazepine) Antidepressant (St John's wort)	SSRI (sertraline), caffeine, beta blockers
Antianxiety agent (diazepam) Antidepressants (citalopram, moclobemide)	Anticonvulsant agent (carbamazepine) Corticosteroid (prednisone)	SSRI (fluoxetine), non-steroidal anti-inflammatory drug (indomethacin), proton pump inhibitor (omeprazole)

Hepatic first-pass effects
Drugs that are predominantly metabolised in the liver can be problematic when administered orally. Drugs absorbed from the stomach and small intestines enter the hepatic portal vein and are transported through the liver before entering the systemic circulation. As they pass through the liver they are subjected to significant metabolism such that the amount entering the systemic circulation is very low, sometimes less than 10% of the original dose administered. The degree of metabolic drug loss is called the hepatic first-pass effect. Therefore, the oral dose may need to be significantly higher than that required for parenteral administration.

Liver impairment
Impaired liver function affects drug metabolism and can result in increased effects. As we age, there is a decrease in efficiency of the liver processes such that the elderly may experience stronger or more prolonged drug

effects when they receive standard adult doses. An adjustment in dosage or frequency of administration may be required for these patients. Some examples of common psychotropic medications that require an adjustment of dosage when used in the elderly are provided in Table 2.4.

TABLE 2.4 – SOME EXAMPLES OF DRUGS REQUIRING DOSAGE ADJUSTMENT IN THE ELDERLY		
Medication	Standard adult doses	Recommended doses for the elderly
Diazepam, antianxiety agent	5–40 mg daily	2 mg bd or half adult dose
Temazepam, hypnotic	10–30 mg daily	10 mg daily
Amitriptyline, antidepressant	75 mg daily	50 mg daily
Imipramine, antidepressant	Up to 25 mg tds	10 mg daily
Haloperidol, antipsychotic agent	1–5 mg daily	1–3 mg daily
Risperidone, antipsychotic agent	4–6 mg daily	1–2 mg bd

Drug excretion
Drug elimination can occur via a number of routes, but the most important are excretion through the kidneys and via the bile secreted into the gastrointestinal tract. Drugs can be eliminated in an unchanged form from that originally administered or after significant metabolism.

Renal impairment
Renal impairment can reduce the rate of drug excretion, resulting in stronger drug effects and/or prolonged action. The elderly also experience reduced renal function that may alter their responsiveness to drugs. Drug dose and frequency of administration may be need to be adjusted in these patients.

The relationship between the rate of drug excretion and drug dosage is quantifiable clinically. The clearance of drugs from the body is strongly correlated to the excretion through the kidneys of a waste product of muscle metabolism called creatinine. Creatinine clearance is used as a clinical indicator of whether it is necessary to alter the drug dose rate in renal impairment. Poor creatinine clearance indicates that drug dosage and/or frequency of administration may require reassessment.

PHARMACOGENETICS

As stated above, metabolic processes are driven by enzymes. These are proteins whose synthesis is programmed by genes. Variations in genetic make-up can greatly affect the presence or amount of enzymes available for drug metabolism. Too much enzyme can lead to faster drug metabolism and elimination. Inadequate enzyme levels can lead to poor metabolism and prolonged drug action.

Thus, the population can be distributed across a continuum representing the effectiveness of drug metabolism. Individuals can be grouped according to whether they are poor, normal or extensive metabolisers. Poor metabolisers will experience higher than expected blood drug levels, which can lead to relatively stronger, possibly toxic, effects and more prolonged action. Extensive metabolisers will eliminate the drug faster than expected leading to lower and shorter lived drug effects. Simple, accurate and quick tests of an individual's genetic characteristics that will indicate their enzyme status are now available or are being developed. These will help to determine the suitability of treatments with drugs whose metabolism is dependent on particular enzyme systems, such as the CYP group.

In some cases altered drug metabolism can be predicted for particular ethnic groups, so that health professionals might anticipate poor or ultra-rapid drug metabolism or faster onset of action for particular psychotropic agents (see Table 2.5). As one of the examples provided in the Table, an African or Arab person is more likely to metabolise a phenothiazine antipsychotic agent, such as chlorpromazine, more quickly than a Caucasian person. Moreover, a person from East Asia is more likely to have a slower onset of action during treatment with the antidepressant drug paroxetine than a Caucasian or someone of African descent.

CONCLUSIONS

This chapter provided an overview of how the brain is organised and how it processes information in order to assist you to understand how psychotropic drugs work. Pharmacodynamics and pharmacokinetics were also discussed, followed by a brief introduction to pharmacogenetics. This information will provide a good basis for the following six chapters.

TABLE 2.5 – DRUG METABOLISM AND ETHNICITY

Genetic variant	Examples of psychotropic drugs affected	Caucasians affected, %	Arabs affected, %	Africans (or of African descent) affected, %	East Asians affected, %
Ultra-rapid metabolisers of CYP2D6-dependent drugs	Phenothiazine antipsychotics A number of antidepressants	5	20–30	20–30	Not determined
Poor metabolisers of CYP2C19-dependent drugs	Tricyclic antidepressant, imipramine SSRI, citalopram Many benzodiazepines	3	Not determined	18.5	14–17
Mutation in 5-HT transporter (resulting in rapid uptake and faster drug response)	SSRI, paroxetine	45–55	Not determined	70	17

SSRI: selective serotonin reuptake inhibitor.
(Adapted from Jones D S, Perlis R H 2006 Pharmacogenetics, race and psychiatry: Prospects and challenges. Harvard Review of Psychiatry 14:92–108)

Recommended reading

Bullock S, Manias E, Galbraith A 2007 Fundamentals of Pharmacology, 5th edn. Prentice-Hall, Sydney

Damasio A 2000 The Feeling of What Happens: Body, Emotion and the Making of Consciousness. Vintage, London

Greenfield S 2000 The Private Life of the Brain. Penguin, London

Kandel E R, Schwartz J H, Jessell T M 1995 Essentials of Neural Science and Behaviour. McGraw-Hill, New York

Teaching and learning activities

1. Name one function of each of the following brain regions:
   a. Cerebellum
   b. Thalamus
   c. Brain stem
   d. Cerebral cortex
2. Define a synapse and state its component parts.
3. Outline the steps associated with the process of neurotransmission.
4. Name two major neurotransmitters and indicate what condition might arise if the activity of each one was altered (note also the direction of the change in the neurotransmitter levels).
5. For each of the following indicate the likelihood that the drug will cross the blood–brain barrier and enter the brain:
   a. Drug A is a large molecule
   b. Drug X is in an uncharged state in the blood
   c. Drug F has affinity for a brain amino acid transporter system
6. Burt Keyborsk is a 42-year-old man with schizophrenia who has developed acute hepatitis C. He has been receiving treatment with the phenothiazine antipsychotic agent chlorpromazine for some time and it has been effective in managing his condition. You observe the onset of extrapyramidal motor disturbances, hypotension and antimuscarinic effects.
   a. How do you account for this alteration in drug effects?
   b. What would you expect to find if you have his blood drug levels checked?

Unit 2
Major Groups of Psychotropic Medications

CHAPTER 3

MEDICATIONS USED FOR DISTURBANCES OF COGNITION AND PERCEPTION

Objectives

The information in this chapter will assist you to:

» Identify the clinical features of two common disturbances of cognition and perception
» Describe the pathophysiology of schizophrenia and Alzheimer's dementia
» Outline the pharmacology of antipsychotic and acetylcholinesterase inhibitor medications
» Understand consumer perspectives and experiences of taking antipsychotic medications and carer perspectives of dementia
» Outline prescribing and administration issues for antipsychotic and acetylcholinesterase inhibitor medications

Key terms and abbreviations

Delusions
Hallucinations
Psychosis
5-HT$_2$ receptors – serotonin receptors
APP – amyloid precursor protein
CPK – creatine phosphokinase

D$_{1-5}$ receptors – dopamine receptor types $_{1-5}$
EPSE – extra-pyramidal side effect
NMDA receptor – N-methyl-D-aspartate receptor
NMS – neuroleptic malignant syndrome

INTRODUCTION

Cognition and perception are processes of the brain that determine how we think, feel and communicate. These processes encompass consciousness, language, sensory processing, attention, memory, judgments and decision making, as well as social interactions. Our emotional states have a significant role in influencing these processes.

Normal cognition and perception are dependent on interplay between the cortical areas and other brain regions including the thalamus, amygdala, hypothalamus, brain stem and corpus striatum. The roles of each brain region involved are summarised in Figure 3.1. Major disturbances of cognition and perception in a mental health context include dementia, delirium, psychosis and attention deficit/hyperactivity disorders. In this chapter, we focus on dementia and psychosis. Attention deficit/ hyperactivity is discussed in Chapter 7.

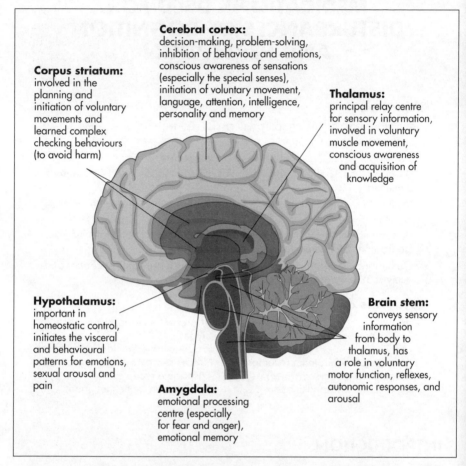

Figure. 3.1 – Roles of selected brain regions in cognition and perception.
Adapted from Human Anatomy and Physiology (7th edn), 2007, by E N Marieb and K Hoehn, Pearson-Benjamin Cummings, Fig 12.12, p 445, with permission.

Disturbances in cognition and perception occur as a result of poor or inappropriate interplay between these key brain regions and are associated with a combination of genetic and environmental factors. The environmental factors include systemic metabolic disruptions, brain infections, substance misuse, changes in nerve membrane thresholds, the formation of scar tissue in the brain, as well as the degeneration or remodelling of nerve pathways.

These disorders can also be characterised by chemical imbalances in neurotransmitter systems. The conceptualisation of these imbalances is often based on an over-simplification of the underlying pathophysiology and is found to be inadequate in explaining some aspects of the disease state; nevertheless, this approach can be used to form hypotheses to provide a rationale for drug development. Chemical imbalances in serotonergic, glutamatergic, adrenergic and/or dopaminergic pathways have been implicated in cognitive and perceptual disorders.

The clinical manifestations of these disorders vary from condition to condition but often involve deficits in:

- language (aphasia, poverty of speech or disorganised speech)
- memory (loss of short- or long-term memory, loss of recall, inability to learn new information)
- attention (difficulty in sustaining, shifting or focusing attention)
- perception (hallucinations, inability to recognise objects, delusions)
- executive function (impairments in planning, judgment, abstract thought)
- social interaction (social withdrawal, apathy about appearance, poor self-esteem)
- affect (flat affect, irritability and agitation).

Important representative examples of relatively common conditions that affect perception and cognition are psychosis, focusing on schizophrenia, and Alzheimer's dementia. In order to facilitate your understanding of the medications used to manage each major type of cognitive and perceptual disturbance – i.e. schizophrenia and Alzheimer's dementia – this chapter is divided into two sections. Section 1 discusses medications used to manage schizophrenia and psychosis, and Section 2 addresses medications used to manage Alzheimer's dementia. A brief overview of each of these conditions will be provided. Suggestions for further reading on dementia and schizophrenia can be found in the 'Recommended reading' section at the end of the chapter.

SECTION 1: MEDICATIONS USED TO MANAGE SCHIZOPHRENIA AND PSYCHOSIS

OVERVIEW OF PSYCHOSIS

Psychosis can be associated with a number of disorders and produces symptoms that lead to the person's loss of contact with reality. In psychosis, the perceptual disturbance of hallucinations, along with disorganised thought processes and/or the thought disturbance of delusions, can lead to bizarre or unusual behaviours. In fact, it is often these that signal to others that the person may be experiencing an alteration in their mental health. As indicated by their name, antipsychotic medications are used to manage and treat the symptoms of psychotic mental disorders.

Antipsychotic medications are used primarily for the psychotic disorders schizophrenia and schizoaffective disorder. They are used to a lesser extent in bipolar disorder and major depression, but are also used to treat a wide variety of disorders including those from primarily physical causes such as delirium and substance-induced psychosis. See Box 3.1 for an overview of the types of mental health problems where psychosis is a major feature. Other uses for antipsychotics include sedation and management of agitation and aggression, reduction of anxiety and as antiemetics (some older/first generation agents such as chlorpromazine and trifluoperazine).

BOX 3.1 – MENTAL HEALTH PROBLEMS WHERE PSYCHOSIS IS A MAJOR FEATURE

» Schizophrenia
» Schizo-affective disorder
» Schizophreniform disorder
» Bipolar disorder
» Major (unipolar) depression of psychotic depth
» Delusional disorder
» Brief psychotic disorder
» Substance-induced psychosis
» Delirium

SCHIZOPHRENIA

The term schizophrenia refers to a group of psychotic disorders characterised by disordered and disorganised thought. Schizophrenia affects a person's perceptions, speech, emotions and behaviours and can be associated with significant difficulty in psychosocial and occupational functioning. The course of the disorder can vary, but is generally chronic with acute exacerbations of varying intensity and frequency, some of which may necessitate hospitalisation. Schizophrenia is observed in 1% of the population across all cultures and affects men and women equally. Treatment and management of schizophrenia focus on reducing symptoms, preventing relapse, enhancing recovery and maintaining remission of symptoms over the long term (Burton 2006). The clinical manifestations of schizophrenia are listed in Table 3.1.

Psychotropic medications have an important but not exclusive role in the treatment and management of schizophrenia, with atypical or second generation antipsychotics being the treatment of choice (RANZCP Clinical Practice Guidelines Team for the Treatment of Schizophrenia and Related

TABLE 3.1 – THE COMMON CLINICAL FEATURES OF SCHIZOPHRENIA

Positive symptoms – the presence of unusual symptoms not present in others in the population (most common in the acute phase)	**Negative symptoms** – normal thoughts/behaviours absent or diminished in people with schizophrenia (seen in the chronic phase)
• Delusions • Paranoia • Hallucinations (visual, auditory and/or olfactory) • Disorganised speech • Bizarre behaviour	• Apathy • Social withdrawal • Limited affect • Anhedonia (inability to experience pleasure)

Disorders 2005). Psychosocial strategies and therapies such as cognitive behaviour therapy, social skills training, occupational support and re-training, and family psychoeducation and support also play a significant role in successful management and outcomes of the disorder.

PATHOPHYSIOLOGY OF SCHIZOPHRENIA

The pathophysiology of schizophrenia remains poorly understood. Susan Greenfield (2000) has proposed that the mind of a person with schizophrenia is overwhelmed by sensory inputs so that the boundaries between reality and illusion become blurred. She suggests that the pattern of neural communication controlling brain functions such as attention, behaviour, perception and cognition is sparse, superficial and rapidly changing.

Two pathophysiological processes associated with schizophrenia appear to dominate the literature – a dysfunction in neurotransmission and abnormal brain structure. The dysfunction in neurotransmission is thought to involve an increase in dopaminergic activation associated with the mesocorticolimbic pathway. The mesocorticolimbic pathway has its origins in the midbrain, a part of the mesencephalon. It projects to brain regions (i.e., cortex and limbic system) involved in the control of behaviour and emotions: amygdala, hippocampus, prefrontal cortex, anterior caudate nucleus and cingulate gyrus (see Fig 3.1). The excess of dopaminergic activity in this pathway in affected individuals is called the dopamine hypothesis of schizophrenia.

Altered brain structure has also been reported in the brains of people who have schizophrenia. Medial percentage regional volume reductions have been reported affecting the whole brain, amygdala and hippocampal regions, as well as the frontal and temporal lobes and their thalamic relays (Halliday 2001, Lawrie & Abukmeil 1998). Moreover, these reviews report ventricular enlargement as a common structural change in schizophrenia. Mitchell and Crow (2005) reviewed the evidence that a decreased level of normal brain lateralisation also plays a role in the pathophysiology of schizophrenia. They argued that there is reduced lateralisation of language to the left hemisphere and possibly even a trans-lateralisation of this function to the right hemisphere in schizophrenia. Language deficits are considered to be important characteristics of the symptomatology of schizophrenia. Hand preference, another characteristic of brain lateralisation, is also altered in schizophrenia as more people with schizophrenia are left-handed and mixed-handed compared to 'healthy' people or mental health consumers without schizophrenia (Sommers et al 2001).

Genetics definitely plays a major part in the development of schizophrenia as a family history is considered an important risk factor. It appears that genetic make-up predisposes a person to schizophrenia, but does not determine its onset. There is interplay between genetics, environmental and developmental factors. Factors that have been implicated include gestational brain injury induced by infection (particularly viral infections like influenza), birth complications and malnutrition. Some researchers have posited seasonal effects (a higher risk associated with babies born in winter) as well as poor exposure to sunlight and deficient vitamin D levels as risk factors for schizophrenia (see van Os et al (2005) for a review). However, these hypothesised risk factors remain controversial and subject to keen debate.

A link has also been established between drug use and psychosis. The current view is that, in general, drug use is not causal in psychosis, but that there is a high rate of co-morbidity between the two. However, cannabis use remains a significant risk factor for psychosis (van Os et al 2005). Furthermore, there are poorer outcomes associated when a person with psychosis engages in substance misuse (Gregg et al 2007).

THE PHARMACOLOGY OF ANTIPSYCHOTIC AGENTS

The evidence supporting the dopamine hypothesis of schizophrenia is drawn largely from empirical observations that drugs that reduce the synaptic action of dopamine in the brain attenuate the symptoms of schizophrenia, while drugs that enhance the action of dopamine (such as L-dopa or dopamine receptor agonists used in the treatment of Parkinson's disease) can induce the symptoms of psychosis. However, although the hypothesis has been further validated through the use of imaging studies, it does fall short of explaining the complexity of the disorder (Toda & Abi-Dargham 2007).

Classic/typical or first generation antipsychotics

Centrally acting dopamine receptor antagonists have been the mainstay of antipsychotic drug therapy for decades, since the introduction of chlorpromazine in 1952. At that time, the discovery of drugs with psychotropic effects created a dramatic change in the treatment of psychosis and led to a new era in psychiatry.

At least five sub-types of central dopamine receptor have been identified. They are represented by the nomenclature D_1–D_5 receptors (see Table 3.2). The efficacy of the first generation or typical antipsychotic agents is strongly linked to their affinity for D_2 receptors: the greater the affinity, the more potent the drug. The first generation medications are more effective in treating the positive symptoms of schizophrenia than the negative symptoms. Moreover, direct imaging studies demonstrate that the first generation antipsychotic agents do alter brain structure in schizophrenia, inducing increases in basal ganglia volumes and decreases in the volumes of different cortical regions (Scherk & Falkai 2006).

TABLE 3.2 – DISTRIBUTION AND FUNCTIONS OF DOPAMINE RECEPTOR SUB-TYPES IN THE BRAIN		
Receptor sub-type	**Distribution**	**Functions***
D_1	Most widespread sub-type in the brain: striatum, limbic system, cerebral cortex, hypothalamus and thalamus	Arousal, mood, emotions and behaviour; motor function; reward and reinforcement; learning and memory
D_2	Mainly striatum, limbic system, cortex, hypothalamus, thalamus, pituitary and midbrain	Reward and reinforcement; arousal, mood, emotions and behaviour; learning and memory; prolactin secretion
D_3	Relatively specific to limbic system; also found in midbrain, cerebellum, hippocampus, temporal lobe and hypothalamus	Inhibits locomotion; emotions and cognition; prolactin secretion
D_4	Frontal cortex, amygdala, hippocampus, hypothalamus, midbrain and basal ganglia	Emotions, cognition and behaviour; arousal and mood
D_5	Hippocampus, thalamus, cerebral cortex, striatum and midbrain	Emotions and behaviour
*A number of functions occur as a result of synergism between receptor sub-types.		

A major problem with these medications, however, is that there are other dopaminergic pathways in the brain that are disrupted by this treatment. The pathways affected are an extrapyramidal system tract that modulates voluntary muscle movements and a hypothalamic–pituitary connection that regulates hormone secretion.

The motor disturbances or extrapyramidal side effects (EPSEs) that can be induced by antipsychotic medication are of four types (see Table 3.3 for an outline of EPSE symptoms and treatment):

• dystonia
• pseudoparkinsonism
• akathisia
• tardive dyskinesia.

TABLE 3.3 – MOTOR DISTURBANCES ASSOCIATED (PRIMARILY) WITH FIRST GENERATION ANTIPSYCHOTIC AGENTS		
Motor disturbance	**Description**	**Treatment**
Dystonia	Involves the face, neck, back and upper limbs. Altered muscle tone leads to wry neck (torticollis), spasming of the eye muscles (oculogyric spasm), facial grimacing, arched back and limb spasticity. Reversible with treatment	Responds to antimuscarinic drug therapy (e.g. benztropine) and by reducing/stopping antipsychotic treatment
Pseudo-parkinsonism	Comprises drug-induced parkinsonian symptoms of tremor, cogwheel and limb rigidity and hypokinesia. Can include slowness of thinking (bradyphrenia) and mental 'clouding'. Reversible with treatment	Responds to antimuscarinic drug therapy and by reducing/stopping antipsychotic treatment
Akathisia	Marked motor restlessness where the person is fidgety, may make rocking motions, walk on the spot and/or pace rapidly. Also includes subjective feelings of restlessness, unease and/or dysphoria. Reversible with treatment	Responds to antimuscarinic drug therapy and by reducing/stopping antipsychotic treatment
Tardive dyskinesia	Involuntary movements of the face, tongue and limbs. Can include lip smacking, tongue writhing, chewing and/or sucking mouth movements, tic-like movements of the eyes and lips, and choreoathetoid (aimless, involuntary) movements of limbs. Often irreversible	If detected early and medication reduced or ceased, may be fully reversible. But usually does not respond to drug treatment and may not respond to reducing/stopping antipsychotic treatment. Prevention is most effective

In general, the greater an antipsychotic medication's affinity for the D_2 receptor, the greater the likelihood of EPSEs (Therapeutic Guidelines: Psychotropic 2003). The more acute EPSEs (i.e. dystonia, akathisia and pseudoparkinsonism) can present anywhere between 24–48 hours (dystonia) and a few days–weeks (pseudoparkinsonism) following commencement of medication (Gray & Gournay 2000). Tardive dyskinesia, a chronic and often irreversible EPSE, usually presents over a longer period of time, months–years after the commencement of medication (Therapeutic Guidelines: Psychotropic 2003). EPSEs can be some of the most frightening and potentially debilitating and stigmatising side effects of the antipsychotics. As tardive dyskinesia in particular can be irreversible, it is vitally important that clinicians closely attend to early detection and management of these side effects. Refer to Box 3.2 for guidelines on detection and management.

BOX 3.2 – GUIDELINES FOR DETECTION AND MANAGEMENT OF EPSEs

» Routine and regular assessment for EPSEs in both primary and secondary care settings, including questioning client and assessing for EPSE using recognised rating scale/s
» Initial prescription of, or transfer to, second generation antipsychotic medications where possible
» Use of the lowest effective dose possible
» Reduction or cessation of medication where possible, particularly for tardive dyskinesia
» Prescription and administration of antimuscarinic medications to treat EPSE symptoms
» Education, reassurance and support of client and family with regard to any fear, anxiety and distress associated with EPSEs

(Gray & Gournay 2000 *Therapeutic Guidelines: Psychotropics* 2003)

The hormonal imbalance caused by first generation antipsychotic drugs involves prolactin secretion. Dopaminergic pathways from the hypothalamus normally inhibit prolactin release. Treatment with the classic antipsychotic drugs blocks these pathways leading to increased prolactin secretion. Hyperprolactinaemia can result in galactorrhoea (a spontaneous emission of breast milk from the nipple at times other than nursing). It is also associated with gynaecomastia (breast development in males) and menstrual irregularities.

The first generations also interact with and block other receptor types including central histaminic and adrenergic receptors, as well as peripheral muscarinic cholinergic receptors. Common adverse effects of these types of interactions include sedation, weight gain, postural hypotension and atropine-like antimuscarinic reactions (such as blurred vision, tachycardia, urinary retention, constipation and facial flushing). Each of the antipsychotic agents will produce a different profile of adverse effects, which may influence the choice of medication for a particular client (see Table 3.4). There are a number of assessment tools that can be useful in identifying the side effects of antipsychotic medications, particularly EPSEs (see Box 3.3).

TABLE 3.4 – ADVERSE EFFECT PROFILES OF THE FIRST GENERATION ANTIPSYCHOTIC AGENTS				
Antipsychotic agent	Motor disturbances	Hypo-tension	Sedation	Anti-muscarinic effects
Phenothiazines				
Chlorpromazine	2	2–3	3	3
Fluphenazine	3	1	1	1
Pericyazine	1	2	3	3
Thioridazine	1	2–3	2–3	3
Trifluoperazine	3	1–2	1	1
Butyrophenones				
Droperidol	3	1	2	1
Haloperidol	3	1	1	1
Thioxanthenes				
Zuclopenthixol	3	1	3	2

1: Infrequently observed adverse effect; 2: somewhat frequently observed adverse effect; 3: frequently observed adverse effect.

BOX 3.3 – TOOLS FOR ASSESSING ANTIPSYCHOTIC SIDE EFFECTS

AIMS (Abnormal Involuntary Movement Scale) is a tool used widely for consumers taking antipsychotics long term. It particularly assesses the risk of tardive dyskinesia

ESRS (Extrapyramidal Symptom Rating Scale) is a tool used for rating all the extrapyramidal side effects

LUNSERS (Liverpool University Neuroleptic Side-Effect Rating Scale) is useful for assessing side effects and can be self-administered but also used by health professionals to help detect client reactions to changes in their psychotropic medications

DAI (Drug Attitude Inventory) is useful for measuring consumers' feelings and attitudes towards their medication

Atypical or second generation antipsychotics

The nature of the adverse effects associated with the first generation or classic antipsychotics led to the development of the next generation of medications to be used in the management of psychosis. These are known as the second generation, atypical or novel antipsychotic agents. Clozapine, the first of these, was originally developed in 1958 but was withdrawn from the market due to the potentially fatal side effect of agranulocytosis (neutropenia). It was only approved for use 30 years later after a pivotal study demonstrated its particular efficacy for treatment-resistant schizophrenia (Hood et al 2007). In Australia and elsewhere, the risk of neutropenia as a side effect has necessitated that a standard monitoring system (Clozapine Patient Monitoring System) be used for all clients prescribed clozapine. Refer to Box 3.4 for an outline of the monitoring protocol.

BOX 3.4 – CLOZAPINE PATIENT MONITORING SYSTEM GUIDELINES

Registration of client with ClopineConnect® (by individual doctors, pharmacists, clozapine coordinators, centres etc., who must also be registered)

» Client is screened pre-treatment for previous clozapine therapy discontinuation due to haematological adverse events and is ineligible for further treatment if that is the case
» Total white blood cell count (WBC) and neutrophil count assessed for eligibility
» Baseline screening for myocardial damage (including patient/family history of heart failure, electrocardiogram (ECG), measurement of troponin I or T, serum creatinine or creatine kinase MB) as myocarditis and cardiomyopathy have been reported with clozapine
» WBC and neutrophil counts must be done weekly for the first 18 weeks of treatment, and at least every 28 days thereafter. Monitoring also required after cessation of use of clozapine
» Monitoring for cardiac changes during treatment is also recommended

---

(Administered by Mayne Pharma Pty Ltd)

While the second generation medications may interact with dopamine receptors, they also appear to interact with a different set of receptors in order to induce their therapeutic benefits. As a result they are less prone to produce the degree of debilitating adverse effects observed (especially the motor disturbances) when the first generation medications are used, although this can be dose-dependent. A number of the second generation medications have affinity for serotonin (5-hydroxytryptamine or 5-HT) receptor sub-types, particularly antagonism at $5\text{-}HT_2$ receptors, which appears to modulate their extra-pyramidal action at D_2 receptors. Some of these agents have affinity for other dopamine receptor sub-types that may also contribute to their therapeutic action. Interestingly, brain imaging studies have revealed that only thalamic and cortical volumes increase after treatment with these drugs (see Scherk & Falkai (2006) for a review). An adverse effect profile of the second generation antipsychotic agents is provided in Table 3.5. See the Summary box below for essential features of second generations and Table 3.6 for daily dose ranges.

TABLE 3.5 – ADVERSE EFFECT PROFILES OF THE SECOND GENERATION ANTIPSYCHOTICS							
Second generation agent	EPSE	Sedation	Hypotension	Antimuscarinic effect	Weight gain	Hyperpro- lactinaemia	Risk of death in older/ dementia clients
Amisulpride	2	1	1	0	1	2	yes
Aripiprazole	1	2	1	0	1	1	yes
Clozapine	1	3	3	3	3	1	
Olanzapine	1–2	2–3	1	1–2	3	1	yes
Quetiapine	1	3	2	1	2	1	yes
Risperidone	2	2	3	0	2	2	yes
Ziprasidone	1	2	1	1	1	2	yes
0: Not observed; 1: infrequently observed adverse effect; 2: somewhat frequently observed adverse effect; 3: frequently observed adverse effect.							

(Adapted from *Therapeutic Guidelines: Psychotropics* 2003, Rossi 2007)

SUMMARY BOX – ESSENTIAL FEATURES OF ATYPICAL MEDICATIONS

» Efficacy in treating positive symptoms of schizophrenia
» A low incidence of extrapyramidal side effects
» Serotonin receptor subtype 2 (5-HT$_2$) as well as dopamine receptor (D$_2$) antagonism

(Hood et al 2007, p 296)

TABLE 3.6 – DAILY DOSE RANGES OF ANTIPSYCHOTICS

Antipsychotic drug	Recommended daily dose range
First generation	
Trifluoperazine	5–20 mg
Chlorpromazine	75–500 mg
Haloperidol	1–7.5 mg
Second generation	
Quetiapine	300–750 mg in divided doses
Clozapine	200–600 mg in divided doses
Olanzapine	5–20 mg once daily or in divided doses
Ziprasidone	80–160 mg in divided doses
Amisulpride	400–1000 mg before meals, in divided doses
Risperidone	2–6 mg
Aripiprazole	10–30 mg

(Adapted from *Therapeutic Guidelines: Psychotropics* 2003, p 124)

NEUROLEPTIC MALIGNANT SYNDROME AND ITS MANAGEMENT

A particular adverse effect of the antipsychotics is neuroleptic malignant syndrome (NMS). First described in the 1960s, NMS is an uncommon but serious consequence of treatment with antipsychotic medications. Original estimates of the incidence of NMS were as high as 3% but more recent data indicate the incidence is actually somewhere between 0.01% and 2.5%, probably as a result of better diagnosis and more rapid intervention. The mortality rate among those diagnosed with NMS is 10–30% (Chandran et al 2003, Zarrouf & Bhanot 2007). The incidence of NMS is thought to be lower with the second generation antipsychotics versus first generations.

The clinical presentation of NMS can be typical, as described in the

Diagnostic and Statistical Manual of Mental Disorders (4th edn), or atypical. The typical presentation includes hyperthermia (>38°C) and muscle rigidity (known as lead pipe rigidity) plus at least two of the following: diaphoresis, dysphagia, incontinence, changes in level of consciousness ranging from confusion to coma, mutism, elevated or labile blood pressure, creatine phosphokinase (CPK) elevation, tremor or tachycardia. However, atypical presentations have been reported (Strawn et al 2007). The cause of NMS remains unclear but it is thought to be caused by reduced dopamine activity in the brain associated with dopamine antagonists, interruptions in nigrostriatal dopamine pathways or withdrawal of dopaminergic medications (Zarrouf & Bhanot 2007). See Chat box 3.1.

CHAT BOX 3.1 – NMS RISK WITH ANTIPSYCHOTICS
Because NMS can be fatal without emergent diagnosis and treatment, maintain a high index of suspicion for this condition whenever you prescribe antipsychotics. (Zarrouf & Bhanot 2007, p 90) This is an interesting quote regarding prescription of antipsychotic medications. The same applies to administration of course.

Certain risk factors for developing NMS have been identified. Factors such as age, gender and time of year are not correlated. Other factors such as agitation, dehydration, restraint, pre-existing abnormalities of central nervous system dopamine activity or receptor function and iron deficiency are more likely to be associated with NMS. In addition, many cases of NMS have been reported in people with physical exhaustion and dehydration prior to onset, or at times of high environmental temperature (Strawn et al 2007). Other medications, such as antiemetics and sedatives, have also been linked to NMS. The syndrome has also been triggered when people with Parkinson's dementia stop taking or reduce the dose of a dopamine agonist or when they switch from one dopamine agonist to another. A history of NMS is also a risk factor for developing another episode of NMS (Zarrouf & Bhanot 2007). See Table 3.7 for medications associated with NMS.

Treatment for NMS is mainly supportive but outcomes are dependent on swift diagnosis and intervention. The most important and immediate treatment is to cease the offending medication and begin supportive therapy. Supportive therapy includes aggressive volume replacement as most people will already be significantly dehydrated. Correction of electrolyte imbalances is also crucial. In cases where there is extreme hyperthermia, external cooling may be required as the peak and duration of temperature are predictive of morbidity and mortality. Intensive medical care is required and should include careful monitoring for

TABLE 3.7 – ANTIPSYCHOTIC MEDICATIONS ASSOCIATED WITH NMS	
First generation	**Second generation**
Haloperidol	Clozapine
Chlorpromazine	Olanzapine
Fluphenazine long-acting	Quetiapine
	Risperidone

(Adapted from Chandran et al 2003, p 440)

signs of complications including cardio-respiratory failure, renal failure and aspiration pneumonia. Pharmacological treatments include: the administration of a benzodiazepine, such as lorazepam, which can ameliorate symptoms and hasten recovery; a dopaminergic agent, such as bromocriptine or amantadine, which can reverse the parkinsonism in NMS; and dantrolene, a muscle relaxant that is sometimes helpful in cases with extreme temperature elevations, rigidity and true hypermetabolism (Strawn et al 2007). See Box 3.5 for an overview of treatment.

BOX 3.5 – NMS TREATMENT OUTLINED
» Immediately cease the offending antipsychotic » Commence intensive medical care » Correct dehydration and electrolyte imbalance » Monitor for symptoms of cardio-respiratory and renal failure » Consider the prescription and administration of medications such as lorazepam, bromocriptine or amantadine and dantrolene

(Adapted from Strawn et al 2007, Zarrouf & Bhanot 2007)

If a person who has experienced NMS then requires further treatment with antipsychotic medications, it is prudent to wait until 1 or 2 weeks after they recover, begin with a low dose and titrate slowly, and reduce risk factors for NMS where possible (Zarrouf & Bhanot 2007). Just because someone has had one episode of NMS it does not follow that they will develop a further one. See Case study on NMS.

CONSUMER PERSPECTIVES ON ANTIPSYCHOTIC MEDICATIONS

Although there have been numerous scientific studies into the pharmacokinetics, efficacy and side effects of antipsychotic and other psychotropic medications, until fairly recently there has been little exploration of the experiences and perspectives of the consumers who take these medications. The findings from a limited number of studies report

CASE STUDY – NEUROLEPTIC MALIGNANT SYNDROME (NMS)

A 54-year-old woman with a history of bipolar disorder was admitted to an emergency department of a general hospital. Upon admission she had high fever, altered consciousness and urinary incontinence, which had been evident for 3 days prior to the admission. Her treatment had consisted of risperidone (5 mg/day), biperiden (4 mg/day) and lithium (1200 mg/day), which had been prescribed 2 months earlier. Due to extrapyramidal side effects these medications had been altered 2 weeks prior to the admission to risperidone (3 mg/day), biperiden (6 mg/day) and lithium (1500 mg/day). On admission her axillary temperature was 39.5°C, and neurological examination revealed somnolence, disorientation and cog-wheel rigidity. Otherwise her examination was unremarkable. Blood results revealed serum lithium was 0.7 mmol/L, creatine phosphokinase (CPK) level was 791 U/L (normal: 26–167 U/L), leukocytes normal, and blood and urine cultures normal. Chest X-ray and lumbar puncture results were normal. Diagnosis of NMS was made according to DSM-IV criteria with fever, rigidity, altered consciousness, elevated CPK and urinary incontinence.

Risperidone and lithium were immediately discontinued. Intravenous rehydration, as well as nutrition via nasogastric tube, was commenced. Peripheral cooling plus the administration of antipyretics were instituted. Bromocriptine (15 mg/day initially, increased to 30 mg/day) was prescribed and administered. The symptoms of NMS subsided within 17 days and she was discharged home on lithium therapy (600 mg/ day) in euthymia.

• The combination of risperidone and lithium was thought to have been the trigger for the development of NMS in this case. Lithium is thought to increase neurotoxicity and increase risk for NMS during antipsychotic treatment.
• Risperidone is considered to have a greater dopamine blockade than other atypicals.

(Adapted from Kosehasanogullari et al 2007)

a range of personal considerations associated with taking antipsychotics that are useful for informing health professionals and guiding their prescription and administration of this group of psychotropics.

The experience of taking antipsychotics includes both positive and negative aspects (see Comment box below). Some consumers have viewed these medications as providing them with hope for their recovery from their mental disorder, while at the same time acknowledging that the very act of taking the medication reinforces they have a disorder and requires their acceptance of this. In taking antipsychotics, consumers can feel as if they have lost self-control and instead are being controlled by both the medications and others such as family and health professionals who are watching over them and/or administering the drugs (Usher 2001).

Consumers have frequently reported they are not adequately informed about their antipsychotic medication or potential side effects by health professionals, although they have found a therapeutic alliance and positive communication with health professionals about their medications helpful in alleviating concerns (Happell et al 2004, Paton & Esop 2005). Some

---

COMMENT BOX

The only thing is that if you don't have to take these tablets you do feel you're as good as everyone else ... like your mind just works without any treatment ... it really struck at the very heart of my self-esteem ... I felt it was eroding of my self-image and when I took the medication it was more or less saying that I wasn't whole ... it says that I am not perfectly OK in the sense that I know there's something wrong but I don't want to say there is.

(Usher 2001, p 150)

consumers receiving depot antipsychotics have experienced them as less helpful for their symptoms, and associated with more side effects, than oral antipsychotics (Castle et al 2002). Other consumers have found depots to be helpful in stabilising their symptoms and that regular administration provided an opportunity to engage in supportive communication with health professionals and other consumers (Phillips & McCann 2007).

Side effects are an integral aspect of the experience of taking antipsychotic medications, and consumers are often concerned about the impact these will have on their lifestyle and social relationships. The distress associated with side effects can be a significant factor in their decision to stop taking the medication (Usher 2001). Consumers have reported that their symptoms and quality of life were more improved, and they experienced fewer side effects, with second generation antipsychotics than first generations (Castle et al 2002, Chue 2006), and that their satisfaction with these medications also supported their adherence to taking them (Gharabawi et al 2006). See Chat box 3.2 for the results of a study on antipsychotic use in Australia.

CHAT BOX 3.2 – CONSUMER FEEDBACK ON ANTIPSYCHOTICS

In a large study on antipsychotic use in Australia, Castle et al (2002) reported that of nearly 1000 consumers taking antipsychotics:

» There was no significant difference in antipsychotic use by gender
» 54.3% were using typical antipsychotics (24.8% of these as depots)
» 8.3% were using clozapine, 13.3% risperidone and 8.8% olanzapine
» Almost 80% had experienced at least one side effect from oral antipsychotics, although 21% reported no side effects
» The most common side effects were diurnal drowsiness (almost 50%) and anticholinergic side effects (78% on clozapine, 45% on risperidone/olanzapine and 58% on typicals)
» Atypicals, particularly clozapine, were considered more effective by consumers for their symptoms than typicals
» Depots were considered less helpful and were associated with more side effects
» Polypharmacy was common with 52% of participants reporting they used more than one psychotropic medication and nearly 10% taking three or more classes of these drugs

---

PRESCRIBING AND ADMINISTRATION ISSUES FOR ANTIPSYCHOTICS

- Antipsychotic medications come in tablet, liquid, wafer, intramuscular injection (including depots) and/or intravenous form, and attention needs to be given to the intended use, relative cost, efficacy, convenience for the consumer and potential side effect profile associated with each before prescribing.
- Starting at the lower end of the daily dose range and slowly increasing dosage can assist in reducing the impact of adverse effects.
- Establishment of a therapeutic alliance and positive and supportive communication with consumers taking antipsychotics are important for effective assessment and maintenance of their treatment.
- Consumers need to be given adequate written and verbal information and education regarding the uses and potential side effects of antipsychotics prior to prescription and administration.
- Particular attention to regular assessment of side effects, including EPSE (especially tardive dyskinesia), is important.
- Consumers receiving first generation antipsychotics should be particularly monitored for signs of motor disturbance, galactorrhoea, sedation, weight gain, type 2 diabetes mellitus, metabolic syndrome and seizures.
- Consumers prescribed clozapine should be monitored according to the Clozapine Patient Monitoring System.
- Consumers who are suspected of having NMS, or have a previous history of it, need review of their continuing need for antipsychotics. There is a risk of reoccurrence of the syndrome.
- While consumers may be prescribed both first and second generation medications at the one time, the benefits from combination treatment are yet to be determined.
- If changing the client over from a first generation to a second generation, a crossover period of 1 to 2 weeks is generally recommended, where the first medication is reduced slowly while gradually increasing the replacement antipsychotic.
- When discontinuing treatment with an antipsychotic medication, general symptoms including nausea and vomiting, headache and restlessness may occur for a few weeks.
- A number of medications cannot be taken concurrently with antipsychotic medications. Box 3.6 shows contraindicated concurrent therapy while using antipsychotic medication.

BOX 3.6 – ISSUES IN PRACTICE: CONTRAINDICATED CONCURRENT THERAPY WITH ANTIPSYCHOTIC MEDICATIONS

» Phenothiazines or carbamazepine are contraindicated when using clozapine due to the potential for bone marrow depressant effects
» Concomitant use of long-acting depot antipsychotics while using clozapine should be avoided because any bone marrow depressant effects that develop cannot be removed rapidly from the body
» Recommended that clozapine not be used with other antipsychotic drugs
» Avoid combining carbamazepine and clozapine
» Avoid combining risperidone and fluoxetine

SECTION 2 – MEDICATIONS USED TO MANAGE ALZHEIMER'S DEMENTIA

DEMENTIA

Alzheimer's is the most common form of dementia, accounting for around 50–70% of all cases (Black et al 2001). It is estimated that around 220 000 Australians suffer from some form of dementia, with the rate of moderate to severe dementia being 1 in 15 in people aged 65 years plus rising to 1 in 4 in people aged 85 years and older (Henderson & Jorm 1998). Other types of dementia include vascular or multi-infarct dementia (approximately 20% of cases) and a range of other less prevalent dementias including alcohol-related dementia, Lewy body dementia, Creutzfeldt-Jacob's dementia, AIDS dementia complex, Parkinson's dementia and frontotemporal lobar degeneration dementias (including Pick's disease). Often, dementia can result from a combination of these types.

Alzheimer's dementia is characterised by a progressive deterioration in memory, thinking, orientation, comprehension, learning capacity and judgment. The phases of the dementia and the accompanying symptomatology are summarised in Table 3.8.

PATHOPHYSIOLOGY OF ALZHEIMER'S DEMENTIA

The accepted view of the pathophysiology of Alzheimer's dementia is that the disease targets and destroys cholinergic nerves within the limbic system and cerebral cortex (Pallás & Camins 2006). One of the contributors to this cell death is thought to be over-excitation of cholinergic nerve cells via N-methyl-D-aspartate (NMDA) glutamatergic receptor activation. In support of this contention, cerebral glutamate levels have been found to be elevated in people with Alzheimer's dementia.

In the early stage of the dementia the focus of the attack is the hippocampus, an area of the brain involved in the establishment of long-term memory and the access to formed memories. The damage progresses to involve other areas of the limbic system. In the advanced stages, the

TABLE 3.8 – PHASES OF ALZHEIMER'S DEMENTIA		
Stage of dementia	Characteristic brain changes	Clinical manifestations
Stage 1 (2–4 years)	Hippocampus decreases in volume by approximately 25%	Forgetfulness, minor communication difficulties, some impairment in acquisition of new knowledge
Stage 2 (2–10 years)	Deterioration in limbic system, marked decline in acetylcholine in certain neurones, further damage to hippocampus	Increasing difficulties with communication, significant impairment in short-term memory, cannot remember any new information Changes in personality, confusion, anger, sadness, lack of concentration and orientation
Stage 3 (1–3 years)	Damage to 90% of hippocampus, limbic system ravaged, cholinergic neurones in whole cortex attacked	Severe long-term memory loss, loss of capacity to communicate or to function normally. Death ensues

(Adapted from Pallás & Camins, 2006)

frontal cortex, involved in executive functions and personality and language, becomes damaged (Pallás & Camins 2006).

The diagnostic hallmarks of Alzheimer's dementia are histological. The brain of an affected person shows the development of neurofibrillary tangles and amyloid, or senile, plaques (see Fig 3.2). Neurofibrillary tangles lead to the collapse of the cytoskeleton, or internal scaffolding, of neurones that determines the characteristic shape of the cell. The cytoskeleton is formed by a protein-based organelle called a microtubule. Its structure becomes disrupted in Alzheimer's dementia, collapsing into insoluble twisted aggregates inside the cell (Pallás & Camins 2006). Amyloid plaques are hard, insoluble plaques that form extracellularly in brain tissue. They are formed from deposits of a toxic fragment of an integral membrane protein called amyloid precursor protein (APP), which is cleaved by a family of enzymes known as secretases (see Fig 3.3). Some of the cleavage products of APP are non-pathogenic and may indeed be protective against the damage that can be induced by oxidative stress. One fragment in particular, called beta-amyloid, is considered a key constituent of the senile plaques. It cannot be effectively cleared from the brains of those people with Alzheimer's dementia and accumulates within the plaques (Nguyen et al 2006, Pallás & Camins 2006). The formation of these plaques is central to the pathophysiology of Alzheimer's dementia, and their distribution appears to correlate with the degree of cognitive impairment.

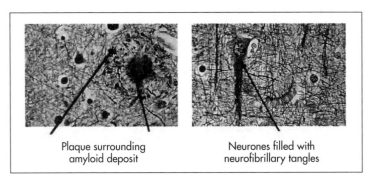

| Plaque surrounding amyloid deposit | Neurones filled with neurofibrillary tangles |

Figure 3.2 – Histological hallmarks of Alzheimer's disease.
Reproduced from Pathophysiology *(3rd edn), 2005, by L C Copstead and J L Banasik, Elsevier-Saunders, Fig 45.1, p 1129, with permission*

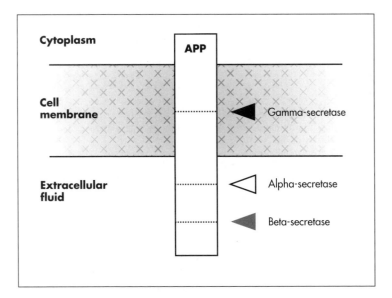

Figure 3.3 – The action of the secretase enzymes on APP
The fragment of APP cut by the beta-secretase enzyme is beta-amyloid, which is a key component of the senile plaques.

The role of genetics in the development of this dementia remains unclear. Genetic predisposition is associated with only 3% of people with

Alzheimer's dementia (Walsh & Selkoe 2004). Gene mutations have been identified in relation to inappropriate APP cleavage and microtubule disruption, and are implicated in the development of Alzheimer's dementia. The presence of a particular gene allele for the synthesis of a lipoprotein called apolipoprotein E is present in a significant proportion of people with Alzheimer's dementia. It is currently considered an important genetic risk factor for the disease because the lipoprotein appears to influence the deposition of APP fragments in the brain (Nguyen et al 2006).

THE PHARMACOLOGY OF DRUGS USED FOR DEMENTIA

At this stage the treatment of Alzheimer's dementia is directed primarily towards relieving the symptoms, with a focus on improving cognitive functioning. The acetylcholinesterase inhibitors have been the mainstay of pharmacological management of the dementia. Recently a novel agent called memantine, belonging to the class of NMDA receptor antagonists, has also become available in this region for use in the treatment of dementia. Memantine appears to slow the cognitive deterioration in moderate to severe levels of Alzheimer's dementia. These drugs have also been referred to as anti-dementia drugs, cognitive enhancers and memory-enhancing drugs (MEDs) (see Chat box 3.3).

CHAT BOX 3.3 – CONTROVERSY REGARDING MEMORY-ENHANCING DRUGS (MEDS)

Dekkers & Rikkert (2007) argue that in Alzheimer's dementia it is the person's 'self' that is being lost, and that the quest for enhancing memory and cognition is one that reduces the human mind down to biological aspects without sufficient attention to broader aspects of 'self'.

Along with researchers, they pose the question: 'What effects do these drugs have on mood, functional status, quality of life, caregiver burden and dementia progression?' and propose that further attention needs to be given to these and other issues before newer generation MEDs are registered for treatment.

Depression can also occur in the middle phases of Alzheimer's and some clients are prescribed antidepressant medications, although those drugs with antimuscarinic adverse effects can amplify cognitive deficits and their use should be avoided if possible. According to Beier (2007), second generation antipsychotic drugs are also useful for psychotic symptoms and behaviours, such as agitation associated with dementia, and are preferable to the first generations due to their higher safety profiles. However, the potential adverse effects (such as sedation, orthostatic hypotension, antimuscarinic anticholinergic side effects and EPSEs) of the second generations may still be a limiting factor when considering their use with this group of clients.

The acetylcholinesterase inhibitors act to prevent the breakdown of acetylcholine in cholinergic synapses, prolonging the action of the transmitter. In effect, the drugs are increasing cholinergic transmission in the brain and enhancing cognition in Alzheimer's patients, and slowing down memory loss. The members of this medication group used in the treatment of Alzheimer's dementia are donepezil, rivastigmine and galantamine. Donepezil is more selective for brain acetylcholinesterase. Common adverse effects (Table 3.9) include nausea, vomiting, diarrhoea, anorexia, dyspepsia, dizziness and myalgia (muscle pain).

TABLE 3.9 – ACETYLCHOLINESTERASE INHIBITORS	
Acetylcholinesterase inhibitor	Daily dose range
Donepezil	5 mg nocte for 4 weeks, increasing to 10 mg if tolerated
Rivastigmine	1.5 mg bd for 2 weeks, increasing to 3 mg bd. Can increase every 4 weeks to 4.5 mg and then 6 mg bd if tolerated
Galantamine	4 mg bd for 4 weeks, increasing to 8 mg bd if tolerated

(Adapted from *Therapeutic Guidelines: Psychotropics* 2003)

There are several problems associated with the use of these drugs in Alzheimer's dementia. A significant number of patients with Alzheimer's dementia do not respond to this therapy and, if they do, the effectiveness of treatment is short-lived (6–24 months). For many patients, the dose needs to be high in order to produce beneficial effects, which leads to a greater degree of adverse effects.

Memantine is an NMDA receptor antagonist that may have a role in counteracting the excitotoxic cholinergic nerve cell death triggered by elevated cerebral levels of glutamate. Under these conditions, the NMDA receptor remains in an activated state allowing prolonged stimulation. Memantine restores the inactivated receptor state, without compromising normal glutamatergic neurotransmission (see Fig 3.4). It is indicated in the treatment of moderate to severe Alzheimer's dementia. Common adverse effects include agitation, insomnia, diarrhoea, vomiting, dizziness and headache. Refer to the Medication in profile box for further information about memantine.

CARER PERSPECTIVES ON DEMENTIA

Unfortunately, due to the progressive effects of dementia on cognitive

A: Activated State

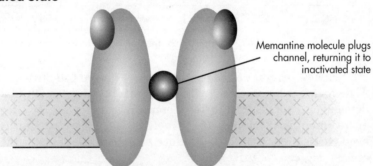

Extracellular

NMDA receptor activated by glutamate and glycine molecules in binding site

Cell membrane

Intracellular

Influx of calcium ions leads to excitotoxicity

B: Inactivated State

Memantine molecule plugs channel, returning it to inactivated state

Figure 3.4 – Proposed mechanism of action of memantine in counteracting excitotoxicity

functioning there is very little research that has explored the perspectives of consumers with dementia. Most of the literature, although this is still quite limited, has focused on carers. Carers, many of whom are family or friends of people with dementia, can experience a range of issues relating to their loved one's condition. One of the most prominent is the burden and distress that can be associated with caring for a person whose behaviour, ability to communicate and interact with others, and performance of daily living activities have deteriorated markedly over time. Studies of carers of people with dementia have found they can experience significant

MEDICATION IN PROFILE – MEMANTINE
Drug class: N-methyl-D-aspartate antagonist
Uses and action: Treatment for moderate–severe Alzheimer's dementia, and can be helpful for vascular dementia. Can slow cognitive deterioration Appears to protect neurones from overstimulation and damage from glutamate transmission and overload of calcium
Daily dose range: 10 mg increasing to 20 mg (maximum daily dose) slowly over 3 week period: 5 mg mane week 1 5 mg bd week 2 10 mg mane & 5 mg nocte week 3 10 mg bd thereafter
Adverse effects: Generally well-tolerated. Most adverse effects mild–moderate severity: dizziness, headaches, constipation, drowsiness, hallucinations
Drug interactions and precautions: Can be administered concurrent with acetylcholinesterase inhibitors Keep dose to 5 mg bd for clients with severe renal impairment

(*Therapeutic Guidelines: Psychotropics* 2003, Robinson & Keating 2006)

psychological distress relating to the behavioural and psychological symptoms such as depression, hallucinations, agitation, irritability and anxiety (Neil & Bowie 2008, Hancock et al 2003, McCarthy et al 1997). Carers have also reported a number of unmet needs in relation to looking after a loved one with dementia, including difficulty managing daytime activities and a need for greater financial assistance to support their carer role (Hancock et al 2003). The grieving process over the deterioration of the person with the dementia, and after their death, has been reported by carers as including difficulty sleeping, feelings of depression and loss of appetite (McCarthy et al 1997).

An important point to note is that carers may well hide or diminish their distress and/or needs in caring for the person with dementia, due to wanting to appear competent and/or be accepted by health professionals. This highlights the need for closer attention and sensitivity by clinicians in assessment of both the person with dementia and their family/carers in order to provide the most effective assistance to them (Neil & Bowie 2008).

PRESCRIBING AND ADMINISTRATION ISSUES FOR MEDICATIONS USED FOR DEMENTIA

- With the prescribing of any psychotropic medication for clients with dementia, doses should start low and be increased slowly as indicated, with regular monitoring for adverse effects.
- Avoid the general use of antidepressants with antimuscarinic anticholinergic adverse effects, as they will counteract the desired action of the acetylcholinesterase inhibitors.
- Avoid the use of typical antipsychotics for Lewy body dementia and Parkinson's disease as they will decrease dopaminergic neurotransmission.
- If benzodiazepines are used (e.g. for sedation or as an hypnotic) they should be restricted to short periods, of no longer than 2 weeks, as they can increase cognitive impairment.
- As acetylcholinesterase inhibitors are expensive, their prescription should be weighed against the likely benefit to the client including consideration of the stage of dementia/level of cognitive decline.

CONCLUSIONS

This chapter has explored medications used to manage psychosis and dementia. These are two major conditions where the primary features are disturbances of cognition and perception. Psychotropic medications play an integral, although not exclusive, role in treating and managing psychosis, and an adjunctive role in managing the symptoms and cognitive decline of dementia. It is important that clinicians understand the pathophysiology and pharmacology of psychosis and dementia, and are aware of the perspectives and needs of consumers and carers where there is psychosis or dementia. Regular and comprehensive assessment of consumers and carers is needed so that effective interventions can be used to reduce symptoms, manage side effects and enhance the wellbeing and quality of life for the person taking the medications, and for the family/ carers who support them.

Useful websites

Alzheimer's Australia – national website providing information and resources and research on Alzheimer's disease, http://www.alzheimers.org.au/

Neuroleptic malignant syndrome information service – http://nmsis.org

Recommended reading

Royal Australian and New Zealand College of Psychiatry (RANZCP) Clinical
Practice Guidelines for Treatment of Schizophrenia (comprehensive overview of
schizophrenia, including psychotropic medication use). Available: http://www.
ranzcp.org/pdffiles/cpgs/Clinician%20version%20full%20schizophrenia.pdf
29 Jan 2008

Wilkinson D 2007 Pharmacotherapy of Alzheimer's disease. Psychiatry 7(1):9–14

Teaching and learning activities

* In your workplace or clinical placement, ask a client or clients taking an
  antipsychotic medication what their experience is of this. What side effects, if
  any, do they have? How do they manage them? What do they consider to be the
  personal benefits or advantages of taking this/these medication(s)?
* Using information from Chat box 3.2 on consumer perspectives on psychotropics,
  discuss the issue of polypharmacy. What implications might the use of multiple
  psychotropics have for the consumer, their family and the health professional
  caring for them? What potential prescribing, administration and monitoring
  issues might there be for health professionals in this situation?

References

Beier M T 2007 Pharmacotherapy for behavioural and psychological symptoms
    of dementia in the elderly. American Journal of Health-System Pharmacology
    64(Suppl 1):S9–S17

Black K, LoGiudice D, Ames D et al 2001 Diagnosing Dementia. Alzheimer's
    Association Australia, Canberra

Burton S 2006 Symptom domains of schizophrenia: the role of atypical antipsychotic
    agents. Journal of Psychopharmacology 20(6):6–19

Castle D, Morgan V, Jablensky A 2002 Antipsychotic use in Australia: the patients'
    perspective. Australian and New Zealand Journal of Psychiatry 36:633–641

Chandran G J, Mikler J R, Keegan D L 2003 Neuroleptic malignant syndrome: a case
    report and discussion. Journal of the Canadian Medical Association
    169(5):439–442

Chue P 2006 The relationship between patient satisfaction and treatment outcomes
    in schizophrenia. Journal of Psychopharmacology 20(6):38–56

Gharabawi G M, Greenspan A, Rupnow M F T et al 2006 Reduction in psychotic
    symptoms as a predictor of patient satisfaction with antipsychotic medication in
    schizophrenia: Data from a randomized double-blind trial. BMC Psychiatry 6:45
    Available: http://www. biomedcentral.com/1471-244X/6/45 29 Jan 2008

Gray R, Gournay K 2000 What can we do about acute extrapyramidal symptoms?
    Journal of Psychiatric and Mental Health Nursing 7:205–211

Greenfield S 2000 The Private Life of the Brain. Penguin, London

Gregg L, Barrowclough C, Haddock G 2007 Reasons for increased substance abuse in psychosis. Clinical Psychology Review 27:494–510

Halliday G M 2001 A review of the neuropathology of schizophrenia. Clinical and Experimental Pharmacology & Physiology 28:64–65

Hancock G A, Reynolds T, Woods B et al 2003 The needs of older people with mental health problems according to the user, the carer, and the staff. International Journal of Geriatric Psychiatry 18:803–811

Happell B, Manias E, Roper C 2004 Wanting to be heard: mental health consumers' experiences of information about medication. International Journal of Mental Health Nursing 13(4):242–248

Henderson A S, Jorm A F 1998 Dementia in Australia (Aged and Community Care Services Department and Evaluation Report No 35). AGPS, Canberra

Hood S D, Orr K G D, Nutt D 2007 Antipsychotics. Psychiatry 6(7):295–300

Kosehasanogullari S G, Akdede B, Akvardar Y et al 2007 Neuroleptic malignant syndrome caused by combination of risperidone and lithium in a patient with multiple medical comorbidities. Letter to the Editor. Progress in Neuro-Psychopharmacology & Biological Psychiatry 31:1147–1148

Lawrie S M, Abukmeil S S 1998 Brain abnormality in schizophrenia. A systematic and quantitative review of volumetric magnetic resonance imaging studies. British Journal of Psychiatry 172:110–120

McCarthy M, Addington-Hall J, Altmann D 1997 The experience of dying with dementia: a retrospective study. International Journal of Geriatric Psychiatry 12(3):404–409

Mitchell R L C, Crow T J 2005 Right hemisphere language functions and schizophrenia: the forgotten hemisphere? Brain 128:963–978

Neil W, Bowie P 2008 Carer burden in dementia – assessing the impact of behavioural and psychological symptoms via self-report questionnaire. International Journal of Geriatric Psychiatry 23:60–64

Nguyen J T, Yamani A, Kiso Y 2006 Views on amyloid hypothesis and secretase inhibitors for treating Alzheimer's disease: progress and problems. Current Pharmaceutical Design 12:4295–4312

Pallás M, Camins A 2006 Molecular and biochemical features in Alzheimer's disease. Current Pharmaceutical Design 12:4389–4408

Paton C, Esop R 2005 Patients' perceptions of their involvement in decision making about antipsychotic drug choice as outlined in the NICE guidance on the use of atypical antipsychotics in schizophrenia. Journal of Mental Health 14(3):305–310

Phillips L McCann E 2007 The subjective experiences of people who regularly receive depot neuroleptic medication in the community. Journal of Psychiatric and Mental Health Nursing 14(6):578–586

Robinson D M, Keating G M 2006 Memantine: a review of its use in Alzheimer's Disease. Drugs 66(11):1515–1534

Rossi S (ed) 2007 Australian Medicines Handbook 2007. Australian Medicines Handbook, Adelaide

Royal Australian and New Zealand College of Psychiatrists Clinical Practice
Guidelines Team for the Treatment of Schizophrenia and Related Disorders 2005
Royal Australian and New Zealand College of Psychiatrists clinical practice
guidelines for the treatment of schizophrenia and related disorders. Australian
and New Zealand Journal of Psychiatry 39(1-2):1–30

Scherk H, Falkai P 2006 Effects of antipsychotics on brain structure. Current Opinion
in Psychiatry 19:145–150

Sommers I E, Ramsey N F Kahn R S 2001 Language lateralization in schizophrenia,
an fMRI study. Schizophrenia Research 52:57–67

Strawn J R, Keck P E, Caroff S N 2007 Neuroleptic Malignant Syndrome. The
American Journal of Psychiatry 164(6):870–876

Therapeutic Guidelines (2003) Therapeutic Guidelines: Psychotropics, Version 5 edn.
Therapeutic Guidelines Limited, North Melbourne, Australia

Toda M, Abi-Dargham A 2007 Dopamine hypothesis of schizophrenia: Making sense
of it all. Current Psychiatry Reports 9:329–336

Usher K 2001 Taking neuroleptic medications as the treatment for schizophrenia: A
phenomenological study. Australian and New Zealand Journal of Mental Health
Nursing 10(3):145–155

van Os J, Krabbendam L, Myin-Germeys I et al 2005 The schizophrenia environment.
Current Opinion in Psychiatry 18:141–145

Walsh D M, Selkoe D J 2004 Deciphering the molecular basis of memory failure in
Alzheimer's disease. Neuron 44:181–193

Zarrouf F A, Bhanot V 2007 Neuroleptic Malignant Syndrome: Don't let your guard
down yet. Current Psychiatry 8(8):89–95

CHAPTER 4

MEDICATIONS USED FOR DISTURBANCES IN MOOD AND AFFECT

Objectives

The information in this chapter will assist you to:

» Identify the clinical features of a range of disturbances of mood and affect
» Describe the pathophysiology of disturbances of mood and affect
» Outline the pharmacology of medications used to manage depression and bipolar disorder
» Understand consumer perspectives and experiences of taking medications used to manage depression and bipolar disorder
» Outline prescribing and administration issues for medications used to manage depression and bipolar disorder

Key terms and abbreviations

Affect
Bipolar disorder
Mood
Serotonin syndrome
5-HT – 5-hydroxytryptamine (serotonin)
GABA – gamma-aminobutyric acid
MAOIs – monoamine oxidase inhibitors (antidepressants)
NA – noradrenaline

NSAIDs – non-steroidal anti-inflammatory drugs
RIMAs – reversible inhibitors of MAO-A
SARIs – serotonin antagonists/re-uptake inhibitors
SNRIs – selective noradrenaline reuptake inhibitors
SSRIs – selective serotonin reuptake inhibitors
TCAs – tricyclic antidepressants

INTRODUCTION

Normal mood and affect is the product of complex interplay between cortical areas (especially the prefrontal cortex and cingulate gyrus) and the limbic system (particularly the amygdala, nucleus accumbens and hippocampus), as well as the hypothalamus and brain stem.

Across the Western world, mental health problems where mood and affect are major features (i.e., depression, mania and bipolar disorder) are highly prevalent and persistent and are associated with significant disability. While bipolar disorder and major depression are considered the more severe conditions associated with disturbances in mood and affect, other conditions of lesser intensity include cyclothymia and dysthymia. Perinatal mood disorders, including ante- and postnatal depression and puerperal psychosis, are also considered to be within the scope of disturbances in mood and affect and will be explored in further detail in Chapter 7. See Table 4.1 for an overview of the features of major disturbances in mood and affect.

As discussed in previous chapters, the management of any mental health problem needs to address the individual's overall situation

TABLE 4.1 – MAJOR DISTURBANCES IN MOOD AND AFFECT	
Disturbance in mood and affect	Features and symptoms
• Bipolar affective disorder	A major psychotic disorder that includes episodes of mania (elevated, expansive mood) and depression that can be of psychotic depth. Mixed episodes with both manic and depressed symptoms can also occur. Usually requires treatment with psychotropic medications
• Cyclothymia	A less severe mood disorder involving chronic fluctuation in mood, with episodes of hypomania (below mania) and depression that are not of psychotic depth. Does not necessarily involve treatment with psychotropic medications
• Dysthymia	A less severe form of depression where the person has a chronically depressed mood for most days for at least a 2-year period. No symptoms of psychosis. May not require treatment with psychotropic medication
• Major depression	Involves one or more episodes of moderate to severe depression that may be of psychotic depth, but no history of manic episodes. Main symptoms include depressed mood, lack of interest in pleasure (anhedonia), significant weight loss or gain, insomnia or hypersomnia, fatigue, feelings of worthlessness or guilt, reduced concentration, recurring thoughts of death and/or suicide. Usually requires treatment with psychotropic medication
• Postnatal depression (PND)	A form of major depression that can emerge within the first few weeks after delivery and up to six months after. PND can last for more than 2 years. Can require treatment with psychotropic medication
• Peurperal psychosis (PP)	This is a less prevalent form of mood disorder that can be experienced by some women post-delivery. Usually includes features of mania and/or depression and psychosis. The onset of PP is sudden and within 2 weeks of delivery. Usually requires treatment with psychotropic medications

and health care needs and, therefore, will usually include a range of treatment options where medication is one of a number of strategies. For moderate–severe disturbances of mood and affect, antidepressant medication and/or medications used to manage bipolar disorder are usually first-line treatments and often need to be taken on a continuing or long-term basis to prevent further episodes. However, medication is a strategy that can be offered in combination with individual and/or group therapies (e.g. cognitive-behaviour therapy), skills training (e.g. assertiveness training, stress and/or anxiety management techniques) and/or lifestyle changes including alcohol reduction, nutritional diet and regular exercise. This comprehensive approach generally provides the most effective management. If medication and/or other therapeutic options are not effective, somatic therapies such as electro-convulsive therapy or transcranial magnetic stimulation, particularly for treatment-resistant depression and/or acute suicidality, may be required.

In disturbances of mood and affect of mild–moderate intensity, psychotherapeutic counselling is often sufficient, and/or the client may choose to use counselling over medication or choose to manage their mood disturbances with lifestyle changes, skills training and/or other approaches including complementary and alternative medicines/therapies.

DEPRESSION

Depression is characterised by symptoms that include intense sadness or loss of interests, along with fatigue, insomnia, changes in body weight, psychomotor agitation, feelings of worthlessness and suicidal intent. Depression is rated as one of the leading causes of non-fatal disease burden worldwide (AIHW 2006, Moussavi et al 2007). Indeed, in 1996 the Harvard School of Public Health projected that depression will become the second leading cause of disease burden after heart disease (cited in Moussavi et al 2007).

It is common, and indeed has been determined to be significantly more likely, for people with other chronic illnesses, such as heart and vascular disease, arthritis and asthma, to have co-morbid depression (AIHW 2006, Moussavi et al 2007). The degree of disability associated with depression is considered to be greater than that of arthritis, asthma, diabetes or angina and is believed to be associated, at least in part, with a poorer level of treatment relative to these physical disorders (Moussavi et al 2007, Andrews & Titov 2007). Depression is also significantly co-morbid with substance use disorders (e.g., alcohol misuse/dependence) and anxiety, and treatment and management of depression will often need to include assessment and management of these related conditions.

BIPOLAR DISORDER

Recent statistics from the USA have indicated that the 12-month prevalence of bipolar disorder is 2% of the population (Grant et al 2005). In bipolar disorder, people experience episodes of mania that alternate with periods of depression. For some consumers with bipolar disorder, there are more episodes of depression; for others, there are more episodes of mania. The symptoms of mania include euphoria or irritability accompanied by insomnia, impulsiveness, talkativeness, grandiose ideas, racing thoughts and ideas, distractability, increased sexual drive and increased motor activity.

In a recent review, Miklowitz and Johnson (2006) reported that bipolar disorder has a lifetime prevalence of around 4% and that it is equally likely to develop in men and women. However, women report more episodes than men. The first episode tends to manifest in adolescents and young adults and, like depression, bipolar disorder is highly likely to be co-morbid with other conditions such as anxiety disorders and substance abuse. Bipolar disorder is also associated with higher rates of suicide than any other mental health problem.

PATHOPHYSIOLOGY OF DISTURBANCES IN MOOD AND AFFECT

The noted British peer and pharmacologist, Susan Greenfield (2000), has articulated a useful perspective on the minds of people with mood disorders. In her book, *The Private Life of the Brain*, she suggests that people with depression become locked in highly personalised inner worlds that are colourless and muffled, where the outside world has less impact. For them, memories and events have exaggerated meanings and significance and this is correlated neurobiologically with neuronal associations, or circuits, that are overdeveloped and overused. People with mania become trapped in the present, overreactive to the outside world, readily distracted and hyperactive. She suggests that it is once again a problem of inappropriately sized neuronal networks. This time they are too modest. In bipolar disorder, when these networks are too small a compensation intervenes so that they rebound to become over-extensive, inducing depression, and then over-adjust back to being too small again.

The accepted conceptual framework used to explain disturbances in mood and affect and provide a rationale for treatment with medication revolves around the biogenic amine hypothesis. It is proposed that these altered mood states are associated with an imbalance in the activity of the biogenic amine transmitter systems involving serotonin (5-HT), dopamine and noradrenaline (NA). In depression, the sensitivity of postsynaptic receptors is decreased, while in mania the sensitivity is elevated (see Fig 4.1). This hypothesis can also be used to explain how a person can cycle between depression and mania in bipolar disorder through changing sensitivities of these transmitter–receptor systems.

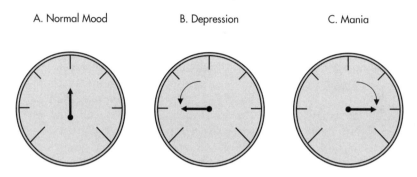

Figure 4.1 – A simple representation of the biogenic amine hypothesis
The dial face represents the activity of the biogenic amine transmitter systems (serotonin, noradrenaline and dopamine) within the brain. To the left of centre the activity is decreased, while to the right it is enhanced. A. The sensitivity of the system is within the normal range. B. In depression, the sensitivity of these systems is lower than normal. C. In mania, the sensitivity of the systems is higher than normal.

The hypothesis is particularly useful in providing a rationale for the development of suitable medications to be used for the management of these disturbances – in clinical trials putative therapeutic agents must be able to demonstrate an effect on these transmitter systems to be considered useful in the clinic.

Clearly, disturbances of mood and affect do not develop simply by altering synaptic transmitter levels. Antidepressant medications can alter synaptic transmitter levels relatively quickly after treatment commences, yet the clinical benefits of this therapy are not observed for another 2–6 weeks. It is argued that changes in receptor sensitivity and neuronal connectivity account for this delay. In other words, brain pathways associated with mood may well be undergoing rewiring.

Recent research has indicated that endocrine and neurogenic factors may have significant pathophysiological roles to play in the development

COMMENT BOX – ANTIDEPRESSANTS

The clinical benefits of antidepressant medications are not usually apparent for 2–6 weeks after commencing medication.

of these mood disorders. A loss of negative feedback control on the hypothalamic–pituitary–adrenal gland axis is considered a hallmark neuroendocrine marker in depression, leading to elevated release of corticotrophin-releasing hormone and glucocorticoids (Maletic et al 2007). Chronic stress or elevated glucocorticoid levels can lead to a loss of neurones within, and a decrease in volume of, the hippocampus. The hippocampus has a major role in the formation of, and access to, long-term memories and contributes in the control of emotions and behaviour. The hippocampus has connections to the amygdala and prefrontal cortex, areas of the brain that have been strongly implicated in the development of mood disorders. In addition to these areas, the basal ganglia and anterior cingulate may play a role in the pathophysiology of bipolar disorder.

In their review, Milkowitz and Johnson (2006) summarised the neurobiology of bipolar disorder. They report that dysregulation of the prefrontal cortex (shown to have a smaller than average volume in people with bipolar disorder), amygdala, hippocampus, basal ganglia and anterior cingulate causes a person who is manic to be less sensitive to negative stimuli, usually associated with threatening cues, and that increased reward motivation may be associated with hyperactivity of the basal ganglia. The brain regions involved in mood disorders are represented in Figure 4.2.

Chronic antidepressant therapy has been shown to enhance hippocampal neurogenesis. The increases in synaptic levels of serotonin and/or noradrenaline brought about by treatment are believed to trigger intracellular signalling cascades that regulate gene expression involved in neuronal function and/or morphology. The expression and actions of key neurotrophic factors that might facilitate this neurogenesis are currently being explored. Neurotrophic factors that have been implicated in this process include brain-derived neurotrophic factor (BDNF), vascular endothelial growth factor (VEGF) and cAMP response element binding protein (CREB) (Maletic et al 2007, Warner-Schmidt & Duman 2006). It has also been suggested that there is lateralisation of the control of affect at the hemispheric level, such that conditions that cause dysfunction of the left frontal hemisphere (e.g., a stroke in that region) can result in depressed mood (Shenal et al 2003).

Changes in intracellular signalling are also implicated in the cycling of mood states characteristic of bipolar disorder. For example, the *Wnt* intracellular signalling cascade appears to be disrupted in this condition. Some of the medications, such as sodium valproate, used to reduce the cycling have been shown to act on this cascade (Rosenberg 2007).

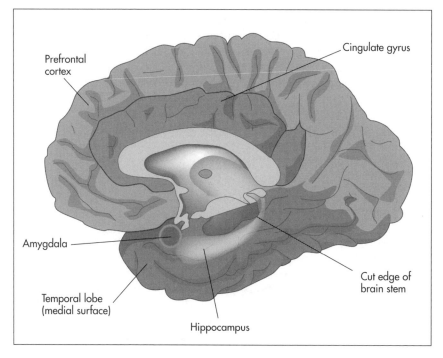

Figure 4.2 – Brain regions implicated in mood disorders.

Functional studies have revealed changes in the size and activity of these brain regions in mood disorders. The integrative connections between these regions may also be disrupted.

Reproduced from Neuroscience: Exploring the Brain, *2001, by M F Bear, M A Paradiso and B W Connors, Lippincott, Williams and Watkins, Fig 18.3, with permission*

PHARMACOLOGY OF ANTIDEPRESSANTS

Ostensibly, antidepressant medications act to raise the synaptic concentration of serotonin and/or noradrenaline. The mechanisms by which the medications can achieve this are by blocking the presynaptic re-uptake pump, inhibiting the enzymic degradation of the transmitter or inhibiting the presynaptic autoregulation of transmitter release (see Fig 4.3). Remember that the changes in synaptic transmitter levels may alter intracellular signalling cascades involved in neuronal function (see previous section). Second generation antipsychotics and antidepressant medications are two of the most commonly prescribed and administered classes of psychotropic medication (Reilly & Kirk 2007), with approximately 5–6% of adults being prescribed antidepressant medication to manage depression and/or anxiety (Mitchell 2007). The major uses of antidepressants are in the treatment and prophylaxis of major depression and the depressed phase of bipolar disorder. Other uses for antidepressants include the management of the anxiety disorders, which include generalised anxiety disorder, obsessive–compulsive disorder, social phobia and agoraphobia, as well for the eating disorder bulimia nervosa and for postpartum depression.

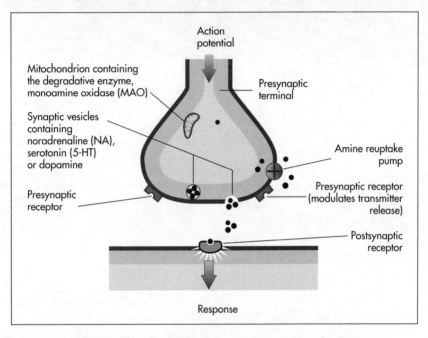

Figure 4.3 – The mechanism of action of the antidepressant medications.
The main target sites and actions for the antidepressant medications are inhibition of the amine reuptake pump, inhibition of the degradative enzyme MAO and blockade of the presynaptic receptor responsible for inhibition of the release of transmitter.
Reproduced from Fundamentals of Pharmacology *(5th edn), 2007, by S Bullock, E Manias and A Galbraith, Prentice Hall, Fig 36.1, p 384, with permission*

The major antidepressant medication groups used in this region of the world are described below according to their mechanisms of action. Generally, due to their tolerability and safety profiles, the prescribing of the newer selective serotonin re-uptake inhibitors (SSRIs) and selective noradrenaline re-uptake inhibitors (SNRIs) has to a large extent replaced that of the older antidepressant groups of tricyclic antidepressants (TCAs) and monoamine oxidase inhibitors (MAOIs). However, the latter two classes of medication are still used for a range of mood-related conditions.

ANTIDEPRESSANTS THAT BLOCK RE-UPTAKE

These medications block the re-uptake of serotonin only, noradrenaline only or both transmitters. For most of these medications the name of the group indicates its action and specificity: selective serotonin reuptake inhibitors (SSRIs), selective noradrenaline reuptake inhibitors (SNRIs), noradrenaline serotonin reuptake inhibitors (NSRIs) and serotonin antagonists/reuptake inhibitors (SARIs). The tricyclic antidepressants (TCAs) block noradrenaline and serotonin reuptake.

The SARI nefazodone acts to enhance serotonergic transmission through two mechanisms: an inhibition of serotonin re-uptake as well as a blockade of presynaptic 5-HT_1 autoreceptors and postsynaptic 5-HT_2 receptors. Common SSRIs, NSRIs and SARIs are listed in Table 4.2, and common TCAs are given in Table 4.3.

TABLE 4.2 – GENERIC AND TRADE NAMES AND DAILY DOSES OF SSRIs, SNRIs AND SARIs			
Generic name	Australian trade names	New Zealand trade names	Daily dose range
SSRIs			
Fluoxetine	Auscap Fluohexal Lovan Prozac Zactin	Fluox Plinzene Prozac	20–40 mg
Sertraline	Zoloft	Zoloft	50–100 mg
Paroxetine	Aropax Oxetine Paxtine	Aropax	20–40 mg
Citalopram	Celapram Cipramil Talam Talohexal	Celapram Cipramil	20–40 mg
Escitalopram	Lexapro	Lexapro	10–20 mg
Fluvoxamine	Flaverin Luvox Movox	N/A	100–200 mg
NSRIs			
Venlafaxine	Efexor Efexor XR	Efexor	75–150 mg

Generic name	Australian trade names	New Zealand trade names	Daily dose range
TABLE 4.2 – GENERIC AND TRADE NAMES AND DAILY DOSES OF SSRIs, SNRIs AND SARIs cont'd			
SARIs			
Nefazodone	N/A	Serzone	300–600 mg

(Adapted from *Therapeutic Guidelines* 2003)

TABLE 4.3 – GENERIC AND TRADE NAMES AND DAILY DOSES OF TRICYCLIC ANTIDEPRESSANTS (TCAs)

Generic name	Australian trade names	New Zealand trade names	Daily dose range
Amitriptyline	Endep Tryptanol	Amitrip	75–150 mg
Clomipramine	Anafranil Placil	Anafranil Clopress	75–150 mg
Desipramine	N/A	Pertofran	100–150 mg
Dothiepin	Dothep Prothiaden	Dopress Prothiaden	75–150 mg
Doxepin	Deptran Sinequan	Anten	75–150 mg
Imipramine	Melipramine Tofranil	Tofranil	75–150 mg
Nortriptyline	Allegron	Norpress	75–150 mg
Trimipramine	Surmontil	Surmontil Tripress	75–150 mg

(Adapted from Birmes et al 2003)

As a secondary action the TCAs block a number of other receptor types: adrenergic muscarinic and histaminic. This accounts for the widespread adverse effects associated with treatment. In overdose the TCAs can induce serious and life-threatening cardiac dysrhythmias. The adverse effects associated with the other medication groups that block transmitter re-uptake are mild and wane as treatment continues. Common adverse effects include nausea, headache, dizziness and insomnia. See Box 4.1 for therapy concurrently contraindicated with antidepressants.

BOX 4.1 – CONTRAINDICATED CONCURRENT THERAPY WITH ANTIDEPRESSANTS

SSRIs should not be used in combination with MAOIs, TCAs, sumatriptan, L-tryptophan.

In general, due to the possibility of adverse events, it is recommended that psychotropic medication, including lithium, anti-seizure medications and non-selective MAOIs, be tapered and discontinued prior to electroconvulsive therapy unless discontinuing medication abruptly would result in adverse effects.

The majority of SSRIs and TCAs are contraindicated during treatment with MAOIs. Transfer between these classes of medication should include a period of between 2 and 5 weeks of ceasing one medication before commencing the other (i.e. an adequate 'washout' period).

Serotonin toxicity is a condition associated with the use of SSRIs, and it arises in approximately 15% of cases where an excess of serotonergic agents has occurred. It is associated with excess serotonin levels and can result from an overdose, an interaction with other medications that enhance serotonin activity or as an adverse effect. Serotonin toxicity is characterised by a triad of clinical features that involve neuromuscular excitation (e.g. hyperreflexia, hypertonia and rigidity), autonomic stimulation (e.g. hyperthermia, tachycardia and sweating) and changes to mental state (e.g. agitation, anxiety and confusion). The severity of toxicity ranges from mild to moderate, through to severe or serotonin crisis (Isbister et al 2007).

Serotonin crisis, also known as serotonin syndrome, is a potentially fatal medical emergency that is specifically due to the interaction of combinations of medications (e.g. MAOIs and SSRIs), and is characterised by multiple organ failure, severe hyperthermia and muscle rigidity (see Case study below). As might be expected, the higher the dose, the more serious the symptoms. These can include agitation, sweating, tremor, hallucinations, tachycardia and shivering. Serotonergic medications that should not be used in combination with SSRIs include MAOIs, sumatriptan, L-tryptophan and the TCAs. The main differential diagnosis with serotonin syndrome is neuroleptic malignant syndrome (NMS), which, as the name implies, is most often associated with the use of neuroleptic or antipsychotic medication. See Chapter 3 for further information on NMS. Other differential diagnoses with serotonin syndrome include delirium tremens (severe alcohol withdrawal), hepatic encephalopathy and central nervous system infections. If appropriate treatment for serotonin syndrome is given promptly, most clients recover completely within 24 hours. Treatment and management of serotonin syndrome are specified in Box 4.2.

Much community attention has also focused on the antidepressant action of the complementary medicine, St John's wort. The consensus

CASE STUDY – SEROTONIN SYNDROME

A 50-year-old man was admitted to hospital with hyperhydrosis, nausea, vomiting and diarrhoea. He had been taking the medications fluoxetine (120 mg/day), meprobamate (400 mg/day) and aceprometazine (13.55 mg/day). The dose of fluoxetine had just been increased.

The client was agitated and had insomnia and hyperreflexia, but there were no focal neurological findings. His vital signs were: blood pressure 155/80 mmHg, pulse 96 beats/min, respiration 20 breaths/min and temperature 37.2°C.

Findings of a full blood count, serum potassium, serum glucose, liver function and renal function tests and erythrocyte sedimentation rate were normal. Blood alcohol test was negative; ECG, chest X-ray, blood gas analysis and cerebral CAT scan showed no abnormalities.

Outcome

The client was diagnosed with a full-blown serotonin syndrome, taking into account the sudden increase in the dose of his fluoxetine and the presence of 3 major symptoms – elevated mood, hyperhydrosis, hyperreflexia – and 2 minor symptoms – insomnia, diarrhoea.

The syndrome was managed by discontinuing his medication. In addition, 3 L of electrolyte solution were administered every 24 hours, 10 mg of IV metoclopramide dihydrochloride every 8 hours and 20 mg of dipotassium clorazepate orally every 12 hours.

The client's nausea, vomiting, sweating and diarrhoea disappeared within 72 hours. His anxiety dissipated more slowly. He was discharged 5 days later.

(Adapted from Birmes et al 2003)

BOX 4.2 – TREATMENT AND MANAGEMENT OF SEROTONIN SYNDROME

» Serotonergic medication is discontinued.
» If in hospital, intravenous electrolytes are usually administered to maintain diuresis.
» Benzodiazepines can be administered for anxiety and agitation.
» Reduction of hyperthermia, use of anti-seizure medication and antihypertensives may be required for severe cases.

is that this plant extract is effective in the treatment of mild–moderate depression. It would appear that there are a number of bioactive compounds within extracts of the plant and there is still debate about which ingredient produces the primary antidepressant action. Research has shown that the possible mechanisms of action of the extract include inhibition of the re-uptake of serotonin, noradrenaline and dopamine and a weak inhibition of the degradative enzyme, monoamine oxidase (Butterweck 2003). Treatment with St John's wort is well tolerated by clients, with photosensitivity a common adverse effect. A major concern associated with treatment is the possibility of drug interactions with other therapies, especially the likelihood of serotonergic syndrome when taken with other medications that enhance serotonergic neurotransmission. It can also interact with warfarin and oral contraceptives.

ANTIDEPRESSANTS THAT INHIBIT TRANSMITTER BREAKDOWN

This group of medications inhibits mitochondrial monoamine oxidase (MAO) in the presynaptic terminal, which is responsible for breaking down any excess transmitter after re-uptake. The inhibition of this enzyme results in larger quantities of transmitter being released during nerve stimulation. These medications are called MAO inhibitors (MAOIs).

There are two subclasses of this group: non-selective and irreversible MAOIs (the classic or older MAOIs) and the newer reversible and selective inhibitors of MAO. There are two isoforms of the MAO enzyme: MAO-A and MAO-B. The MAO-A isoform accounts for approximately one-third of the MAO present in the brain and is widespread throughout the periphery. It plays a significant role in the metabolism of serotonin and noradrenaline. MAO-B is the primary isoform in brain and liver and is more involved in the breakdown of dopamine. The newer MAO inhibitors are more selective for MAO-A and bind reversibly to the enzyme. These medications are therefore called the reversible inhibitors of MAO-A (RIMAs). Common agents in this category are listed in Table 4.4.

TABLE 4.4 – GENERIC AND TRADE NAMES AND DAILY DOSES OF MONOAMINE OXIDASE INHIBITORS (MAOIs)			
Generic names	Australian trade names	New Zealand trade names	Daily dose range
Non-selective (older)			
Phenelzine	Nardil		45–60 mg
Tranylcypromine	Parnate	Parnate	30–40 mg
RIMA* (newer)			
Moclobemide	Arima Aurorix Clobemix Maosig Mohexal	Aurorix	300–600 mg

*RIMA: reversible inhibitor of MAO-A

As the classic MAOIs are non-selective for these isoforms and inhibit liver MAO activity, effective metabolism of blood levels of the biogenic amines is poor when they are elevated. Under these conditions, dietary triggers of peripheral noradrenaline release can result in a marked overstimulation of the cardiovascular system. Tyramine is an amino acid abundant in a number of foods, particularly fermented foods like cheese and alcoholic drinks. When tyramine enters the body it leads to widespread release of noradrenaline. Under normal conditions, the noradrenaline would be degraded by hepatic MAO before it can induce excessive cardiovascular stimulation leading to an acute hypertensive state and cardiac dysrhythmia. Foods that are rich in tyramine are listed in Box 4.3. These foods need to be excluded from the diet during classic MAOI therapy. This food–drug interaction is called a hypertensive crisis, the 'tyramine reaction' or the 'cheese reaction'. Other antidepressant medications as well as other amine medications, such as cough medications, sinus and nasal decongestants, epinephrine, narcotic drugs, stimulants and medication used to treat hayfever and asthma, also need to be avoided during the use of MAOIs.

BOX 4.3 – EXAMPLES OF TYRAMINE-RICH FOODS

» Processed meats (e.g. salami, bacon)
» Fermented foods (e.g. cheese, especially matured cheese, alcoholic drinks)
» Fruits and vegetables (e.g. avocados, figs, bananas in large amounts, broad beans, soybean paste)
» Pickled foods and cured meats
» Sauces (e.g. soy sauce)
» Stock cubes
» Yeast extracts (e.g. Vegemite)

Due to their relative selectivity for MAO-A, RIMAs do not require dietary restriction. Common adverse effects of the RIMAs include nausea, dizziness and insomnia. For the classic MAOIs, it is common to observe antimuscarinic and antiadrenergic side effects.

ANTIDEPRESSANTS THAT INHIBIT PRESYNAPTIC AUTOREGULATION

This category of action describes the tetracyclic antidepressants. This group is also known as the second generation antidepressants. They act on presynaptic α_2 adrenergic autoreceptors responsible for blocking the release of transmitter into the synaptic gap. This mechanism is present to halt excessive release of transmitter when the nerve is being overstimulated. The tetracyclic antidepressants inhibit the presynaptic α_2 receptors and allow increased release of transmitter. Some of these agents can also block noradrenaline reuptake, further contributing to their antidepressant action. Common agents from this group are listed in Table 4.5.

Common adverse effects of this treatment include headache, drowsiness and fatigue. There is a risk of suppression of bone marrow cells resulting in blood dyscrasias, but this is very rare. Nevertheless, blood tests should be monitored during therapy.

Generic names	Australian trade names	New Zealand trade names	Daily dose range
Maprotiline	N/A	Ludiomil	75–150 mg
Mianserin	Lumin Tolvon	Tolvon	60–90 mg
Mirtazapine	Avanza Axit Mirtazon Remeron	N/A	30–45 mg

TABLE 4.5 – GENERIC AND TRADE NAMES AND DAILY DOSES OF TETRACYCLIC ANTIDEPRESSANTS

CONSUMER PERSPECTIVES ON DISTURBANCES IN MOOD AND AFFECT

In the past decade or so, public stigma and discrimination associated with depression and other disturbances of mood and affect have lessened somewhat, in part due to government initiatives and public campaigns designed to educate the community and de-stigmatise this and other mental health problems. Organisations addressing depression and co-morbid anxiety – such as beyondblue in Australia and the depression website run by the Ministry of Health in New Zealand – are well-regarded and effective resources used by many in the community. Sharing the experiences of depression and other mental health problems of media stars and well known public figures has also contributed to these conditions becoming more accepted, and acceptable, in the community. However, discrimination and stigma related to mental health problems such as mood disturbances remain ongoing concerns for many consumers and require continued preventative efforts.

In this context, there have been a number of studies that have sought to gain the perspectives of people who have experienced disturbances of mood and affect such as depression and bipolar disorder. Some of these have focused on health professionals' own mental illnesses and their experience of stigma, including from their health care colleagues. In an Australian study of 29 nurses, the majority of whom had been diagnosed with depression or bipolar disorder, Joyce, Hazelton and McMillan (2007) reported that, while some nurses experienced positive and supportive responses from health care professionals, most did not feel supported by their co-workers or by nursing staff when they were receiving treatment in hospital. Many of the nurses in the study experienced discrimination, gossip and negative reactions about their mental health problem from co-workers. In terms of experiencing treatment for their mental health problem, the nurses also described their feelings of 'being managed' by medication. One nurse said:

> I don't think drugs are you know the be all and end all but I just know that when I don't take it, I go really psychotic, I mean really, really psychotic and barricade myself in houses and delusional and all the rest so I just take it so that I don't get, yeah, super sick.
>
> (Joyce et al 2007, pp 377–378)

Another explains:

> I have delusions and act on them, which can be very embarrassing. The last episode of illness that I had was I think my medication was too light and … I've just recently changed psychiatrists. He put me on a higher dose. It seems to work better. As I get older I seem to have deeper and darker depressions and more frequent … I guess for me the delusions are the most distressing as well as the depression.
>
> (Joyce et al 2007, p 378)

Hope is an important factor in the experience of depression, as feelings of hopelessness, isolation and despair, and difficulties connecting in relationships with others, are all features of the illness. Consumers have described how they wear a 'mask' of depression, a façade they develop to hide their depression despite this requiring a great deal of effort to sustain. They also explain that the relationship they have with health professionals can be hope-destroying, particularly when the health professional is preoccupied with medication to the detriment of talking with and listening to them (Houghton 2007). While consumers acknowledge the value and importance of medication, this is only one facet of their need for support. One consumer explains how impersonal it can be when the doctor focuses on medication alone:

> … the first thing they do is get the prescription pad. They were treating the symptoms of my illness – they weren't treating Debbie.
>
> (Houghton 2007, p 4)

When the person is listened to by health professionals, however, they can experience this as being particularly therapeutic and feel understood and accepted:

> … Sometimes there is a need to tell your story when the story is one that you feel you cannot tell many people and when you live with a part of yourself that is unknown to most others that you meet or work with. Listening, I was reminded, was more than a bag of skills used in an appropriate order but a real sense of engagement.
>
> (Burnard 2007, p 810)

Consumers have generally agreed that recovery from depression is influenced by a number of factors, of which medication plays an important, but not the only, role. Two-thirds of the 60 consumers in a study by Badger and Nolan (2007) reported that medication had contributed to their recovery and that having a greater sense of control over their medications had contributed to better outcomes. Those who found medication helpful had experienced few side effects and greater improvement of their symptoms, which they attributed to antidepressant medication. Interestingly, two-thirds of the participants also reported they had tried other treatments such as over-the-counter treatments and complementary and alternative therapies such as St John's wort, although only 12 participants found these had contributed towards their recovery. It is also important to note that health professionals such as GPs, community mental health nurses and practice nurses who acknowledged and encouraged consumers' roles in their recovery were experienced as being caring and offering comprehensive care that met the consumers' needs. GPs in particular have an important role to play in the management of depression as they are often the first health professional to assess, diagnose and manage the illness. In one study (Simon et al 2006), 75% of consumers reported GPs as their first contact, with 65% considering that GPs played an essential role in providing information on their illness. All 40 participants in this study acknowledged that the main reason they used psychotropic medication was to gain an improvement in their symptoms (see Comment box below).

COMMENT BOX – SSRIs

I started taking (an SSRI) which convinced me that there was a problem because I felt so much better, the change was fantastic.

(Badger & Nolan 2007, p 29)

PRESCRIBING AND ADMINISTRATION ISSUES FOR ANTIDEPRESSANTS

- Establishment of a therapeutic alliance and attentive listening to and communication with consumers taking antidepressants is important to their overall recovery.
- Consumers need to be assessed for use of over-the-counter and complementary and alternative therapies/medicines before prescribing of antidepressants in order to check for potential drug interactions. St John's wort has particular interactivity with serotonergic antidepressants, notably the SSRIs.
- Consumers need to be given adequate written and verbal information

and education regarding the uses and potential side effects of antidepressants prior to prescribing and administration.

- Consumers should be advised that therapeutic effects for all antidepressants will not be evident for at least 1–2 weeks.
- Consumers taking antidepressants should have regular risk assessment and monitoring for increased suicide risk in the 2–6 week period following commencement on the medication.
- Particular attention to regular assessment of adverse effects from antidepressants, particularly serotonin syndrome with serotonergic antidepressants, is important.
- Clients prescribed SSRIs should be informed of the risk of discontinuation syndrome with rapid stopping or reduction of dose. Clinicians should ensure dosage is slowly reduced over a period of 2 weeks.
- Clients prescribed mianserin may develop neutropenia. All clients on the medication should have a full blood count prior to treatment, repeated every 4–6 weeks and/or if symptoms of neutropenia develop. The medication should be ceased if neutropenia develops.
- Clients prescribed MAOIs should be given written and verbal information on their potential interaction with foods and medication containing tyramine, and informed of the risk of hypertensive crisis and cardiac dysrthymias if guidelines are not adhered to.

CLINICAL ALERT 4.1 – COMMENCEMENT OF ANTIDEPRESSANTS

The clinical benefits of antidepressant medications are not usually apparent for 2–6 weeks after commencing medication.

During this early period of treatment, clinicians need to be mindful that the lack of energy associated with depression may lift while the depressed mood may not, and there is a risk that clients may act on their suicidal thoughts.

Close monitoring and risk assessment of the client during this period is important.

PHARMACOLOGY OF MEDICATIONS USED TO MANAGE BIPOLAR DISORDER

The treatment of bipolar disorder is perhaps more complex than some other mental disorders as it needs to be considered in terms of acute manic, depressed and/or mixed episodes and involves treatment for both psychotic symptoms and mood disturbances, along with treatment for prophylaxis or prevention of further episodes. The depression in bipolar disorder can be more difficult to treat than the mania. Due to the psychotic features that are often present in bipolar disorder, including the depressed phase, treatment can consist of combinations of antipsychotic and antidepressant or mood stabiliser medications (Fountoulakis et al

2007). Refer to Box 4.4 for examples of the main combinations that have been found to be effective.

BOX 4.4 – COMBINATIONS OF ANTIPSYCHOTICS AND ANTIDEPRESSANTS OR MOOD STABILISERS EFFECTIVE FOR THE DEPRESSED PHASE OF BIPOLAR DISORDER
Olanzapine – fluoxetine combination
Quetiapine – lamotrigine combination

(Fountoulakis et al 2007)

There are a number of medications that are useful in the management of bipolar disorder that can control manic episodes, prevent recurrences or inhibit rapid cycling between extremes of mood. These medications include lithium carbonate, the anti-seizure agents sodium valproate, carbamazepine and lamotrigine, as well as the atypical antipsychotic agent olanzapine. With the exception of lamotrigine, the medications are more effective in the control of mania than in the treatment of the depressed phase of bipolar disorder (Thase & Sachs 2000). A further novel anti-seizure medication, topiramate, has been used for bipolar disorder, particularly as treatment for acute mania. However, recent evidence from studies suggests that topiramate lacks efficacy for treating mania, although it may have some efficacy for treating bipolar disorder in the depressed phase. Topiramate has, however, shown strong efficacy as a weight-reducing agent for clients who have gained weight from psychotropic medication and can be useful as adjunctive therapy for clients with bipolar disorder, binge eating disorder, bulimia nervosa and alcohol dependence (Arnone 2005, Kirov & Tredget 2005).

Lithium carbonate is a naturally occurring salt that has been used in the treatment of mania since the discovery of its efficacy by the Australian John Cade in 1949. Even with the later advent of the anti-seizure and other medications useful for bipolar disorder, this medication remains the gold standard in the treatment of all phases of bipolar disorder, although it appears to be more useful for treating mania than depression (Fountoulakis et al 2007). Lithium carbonate primarily disrupts intracellular signalling cascades that result from activation of postsynaptic receptors within the pathways involved in affect, thus stabilising mood. There is also evidence that it inhibits presynaptic release of amine transmitters such as noradrenaline. Common adverse effects include weight gain, sedation, fine tremor, thirst, polyuria and gastrointestinal upset. There is also a fine line between therapeutic blood levels and toxic levels of lithium, and it is potentially quite toxic at high doses, leading to nervous system and renal damage. Treatment should therefore be closely monitored. Long-term treatment may induce a hypothyroid state. Refer to Table 4.6 for blood levels and precautions when prescribing and monitoring lithium use.

TABLE 4.6 – BLOOD LEVELS, PRECAUTIONS AND CONTRAINDICATIONS WITH LITHIUM
Blood levels **Therapeutic** = 0.6–1.2 mmol/L for acute mania 0.6–0.8 mmol/L for maintenance **Toxic** = > 2.0 mmol/L (but toxicity may develop at lower levels, particularly in older clients) This is a medical emergency requiring immediate cessation of the medication, and: • if the level is below 3 mmol/L, use of a saline infusion to encourage diuresis • if the level is over 3 mmol/L or the client is comatose, in shock, or severely dehydrated, renal dialysis needs to be used
Precautions • Blood samples for testing should be taken 12 hours after the last dose when lithium has been taken for at least 5–7 days • Blood levels need to be monitored weekly until stable and then monthly • If the blood level for lithium exceeds 1.5 mmol/L, the next dose should be withheld and the treating doctor notified • Care should be taken with concomitant diabetes, thyroid disorders, history of seizures or urinary retention • Signs of lithium toxicity include nausea, vomiting, diarrhoea, coarse hand tremor, lethargy, ataxia, weakness, drowsiness, dysarthria • High toxicity is characterised by signs of decreased blood pressure, irregular pulse, fever, ECG changes, impaired consciousness, disorientation, seizures, coma and death
Contraindications • Should not be used with concomitant cardiac or renal disease, pregnancy and lactation, or where the person is dehydrated or sodium depleted or has brain damage

(Adapted from *Therapeutic Guidelines* 2003)

The anti-seizure agents stabilise hyperactive brain circuits involved in mania. They are thought to induce these effects through a combination of impaired sodium movement across nerve membranes and an enhanced activity of the primary inhibitory GABA transmitter system. There is evidence that valproate also inhibits the activity of the excitatory glutamate transmitter system (refer to Chat box 4.1 for discussion of a possible link between treatments). Common adverse effects include rashes and gastrointestinal disturbances. Serious adverse effects associated with treatment include elevated liver enzyme levels, Stevens-Johnson syndrome (a severe immune reaction that can be fatal; clinical manifestations include fever, malaise and blistering of the skin and mucous membranes) and depression of blood cells levels, particularly white blood cells and platelets.

CHAT BOX 4.1 – LINK BETWEEN ANTIDEPRESSANTS, LITHIUM AND ANTIPARKINSON MEDICATIONS?

A large pharmacoepidemiological study by Brandt-Christensen et al (2006) found that people prescribed antidepressants or lithium had an increased risk of being treated with antiparkinson drugs (not including antimuscarinic drugs such as benztropine or benzhexol that are used to treat EPSE).

The authors suggested that, according to the 'serotonin hypothesis', disturbances of mood could be viewed as prodromal symptoms in Parkinson's disease due to the effects of decreased serotonin activity prior to the onset of the main symptoms of this neurodegenerative disorder. Therefore, they speculated that treatment with antidepressants or lithium could precipitate Parkinson's disease by interfering with the balance of neurotransmitters in the brain. Another possible explanation was that having a disturbance of mood or anxiety could be a risk factor for the later development of Parkinson's disease.

They concluded that people treated with antidepressants or lithium were at higher risk of developing Parkinson's disease.

Discussion question:

This study is an example of how treatment for one mental health issue may lead to treatment for further or related conditions:

» What implications might this have for prescribing and monitoring consumers taking these medications?
» What impact might this kind of information have on consumers' adherence to these medications?

The second generation antipsychotic agent, olanzapine, can also be used as it acts to block central dopamine receptors and selected serotonergic (5-HT$_2$) receptors. Note that this mechanism conforms to the biogenic amine hypothesis of mood disorders. Common adverse effects include drowsiness, weight gain and hyperglycaemia. When commencing treatment with olanzapine, clients need to be monitored for depressed blood cell counts and severe orthostatic hypotension.

Refer to Box 4.5 for contraindications to medications used to manage bipolar disorder.

BOX 4.5 – CONTRAINDICATED CONCURRENT THERAPY WITH MEDICATIONS USED TO MANAGE BIPOLAR DISORDER

» Lithium should not be used with diuretics, angiotensin-converting enzyme (ACE) inhibitors, neuroleptics, non-steroidal anti-inflammatory drugs (NSAIDS).
» MAOIs are contraindicated when taking anti-seizure medication.
» Carbemazepine should not be used concurrent with clozapine due to the increased risk of blood dyscrasias.

PRESCRIBING AND ADMINISTRATION ISSUES FOR MEDICATIONS USED TO MANAGE BIPOLAR DISORDER

- Medications used to manage bipolar disorder are primarily available in tablet or capsule form.
- Clients need to be informed of the importance of continuing to take their medication as prophylaxis even when they are feeling well and have no symptoms.
- When commencing olanzapine treatment for bipolar disorder, clients should be monitored for depressed blood cell counts and orthostatic hypotension.
- When prescribed lithium, clients should be educated about the need for regular blood tests, the adverse effects and risk of toxicity, and the need to maintain adequate fluid (at least 2 litres) and sodium intake and to replace fluid and sodium after exercising.
- When prescribed anti-seizure medications, clients need to be advised to avoid abrupt cessation of the medication.

CONCLUSIONS

This chapter has explored medications used to manage the major disturbances in mood – depression and bipolar disorder. Antidepressant medications, and medications used to treat mania, play an important although not exclusive role in treating and managing disturbances of mood and affect. For many consumers, medications are used to gain an improvement in their symptoms, often in combination with other psychosocial strategies. It is important that clinicians understand the pathophysiology and pharmacology of depression and bipolar disorder and are aware of the perspectives and needs of consumers who experience these mental health problems. One of the most important and effective interventions is careful listening by the clinician. Regular and comprehensive assessment of consumers and carers is needed so that the most effective interventions can be used to reduce symptoms, manage side effects and enhance the wellbeing and quality of life of the consumers taking the medications and the people who support them.

Useful websites

beyondblue – national website for the Australian national depression initiative, providing resources, research and other information, http://www.beyondblue.org.au/index.aspx?

Depression – national website run by the Ministry of Health in New Zealand,

including phone helpline and information and other resources, http://www.
depression.org.nz/

Recommended reading

Gartside S, Cowen P 2006 Pharmacology of drugs used in the treatment of mood
disorders. Psychiatry 5(5):162–166

Royal Australian and New Zealand College of Psychiatry (RANZCP) Clinical
Practice Guidelines for the Treatment of Bipolar Disorder – comprehensive
overview of bipolar disorder, including psychotropic medication use. Available:
http://www.ranzcp.org/pdffiles/cpgs/Bipolar%20Clinician%20Full.pdf
29 Jan 2008

Royal Australian and New Zealand College of Psychiatry (RANZCP) Clinical
Practice Guidelines for the Treatment of Depression – comprehensive overview
of depression, including psychotropic medication use. Available: http://www.
ranzcp.org/pdffiles/cpgs/Depression%20Clinican%20Full.pdf 29 Jan 2008

Teaching and learning activities

- Consider the comments on medications made by the nurses in the study by Joyce
  et al (2007) in the section on 'Consumer perspectives on disturbances in mood
  and affect'.
- What issues can you see that health professionals who are also mental health
  consumers might experience?
- How might nurses' professional knowledge impact on their acceptance and
  understanding of treatment with psychotropic medication?
- What implications do negative attitudes and stigma about mental illness from
  health care colleagues have for the prospects of de-stigmatisation of the general
  public?

References

Andrews G, Titov N 2007 Depression is very disabling (Comment). Lancet
370:808–809

Arnone D 2005 Review of the use of Topiramate for treatment of psychiatric
disorders. Annals of General Psychiatry, 4(5). Available: http://www.annals-
general-psychiatry.com/content/4/1/5 21 Apr 2008

Australian Institute of Health and Welfare 2006 Australia's Health. AIHW Cat No
AUS 73. AIHW, Canberra

Badger F, Nolan P 2007 Attributing recovery from depression. Perceptions of people
cared for in primary care. Journal of Nursing and Healthcare of Chronic Illness/
Journal of Clinical Nursing 3a:25–34

Birmes P, Coppin D, Schmitt L et al 2003 Serotonin syndrome: A brief review.
Canadian Medical Association Journal 168(11):1439–1442

Brandt-Christensen M, Kvist K, Nilsson F M et al 2006 Treatment with antidepressants and lithium is associated with increased risk of treatment with antiparkinson drugs: a pharmacoepidemiological study. Journal of Neurological and Neurosurgical Psychiatry 77:781–783

Burnard P 2007 Seeing the psychiatrist: An autoethnographic account. Journal of Psychiatric and Mental Health Nursing 14(8):808–813

Butterweck V 2003 Mechanism of action of St John's wort in depression: What is known? CNS Drugs 17:539–562

Fountoulakis K N, Grunze H, Panagiotidis P et al 2007 Treatment of bipolar depression: an update. Journal of Affective Disorders doi:10.1016/j. jad.2007.10.1016

Grant B F, Stinson F S, Hasin D S et al 2005 Prevalence, correlates and comorbidity of bipolar I disorder and axis I and II disorders: Results from the National Epidemiology Survey on alcohol and related conditions. Journal of Clinical Psychiatry 66:1205–1215

Greenfield S 2000 The Private Life of the Brain. Penguin, London

Houghton S 2007 Exploring hope: Its meaning for adults living with depression and for social work practice. Australian e-Journal for the Advancement of Mental Health, 6(3). Available: www.auseinet.com/journal/vol6iss3/houghton.pdf 21 Apr 2008

Isbister G K, Buckley N A, Whyte I M 2007 Serotonin toxicity: a practical approach to diagnosis and treatment. Medical Journal of Australia 187(6):361–365

Joyce T, Hazelton M, McMillan M 2007 Nurses with mental illness: Their workplace experiences. International Journal of Mental Health Nursing 16(6):373–380

Kirov G, Tredget J 2005 Add-on topiramate reduces weight in overweight patients with affective disorders: A clinical case series. BMC Psychiatry, 5(19). Available: http://www.biomedcentral.com/147-244X/5/19 21 Apr 2008

Maletic V, Robinson M, Oakes T et al 2007 Neurobiology of depression: An integrated view of key findings. International Journal of Clinical Practice 61:2030–2040

Milkowitz D J, Johnson S L 2006 The psychopathology and treatment of bipolar disorder. Annual Review of Clinical Psychology 2:199–235

Mitchell P B 2007 St John's wort for depression. Medicine Today 8(2):67–68

Moussavi S, Chatterji S, Verdes E et al 2007 Depression, chronic diseases, and decrements in health: Results from the World Health Surveys. Lancet 370:851–858

Reilly T H, Kirk M A 2007 Atypical antipsychotics and newer antidepressants. Emergency Medicine Clinics of North America 25:477–497

Rosenberg G 2007 The mechanisms of action of valproate in neuropsychiatric disorders: Can we see the forest from the trees? Cellular and Molecular Life Sciences 64:2090–2103

Shenal B V, Harrison D W, Demaree H A 2003 The neuropsychology of depression: A literature review and preliminary model. Neuropsychology Review 13:33–42

Simon D, Loh A, Wills C E et al 2006 Depressed patients' perceptions of depression treatment decision-making. Health Expectations 10:62–74

Thase M E, Sachs G S 2000 Bipolar depression: Pharmacotherapy and related therapeutic strategies. Biological Psychiatry 48:558–572

Therapeutic Guidelines 2003 Therapeutic Guidelines: Psychotropic (5th edn). Therapeutic Guidelines Limited, North Melbourne, Australia

Warner-Schmidt J L, Duman R S 2006 Hippocampal neurogenesis: opposing effects of stress and antidepressant treatment. Hippocampus 16:239–249

CHAPTER 5

MEDICATIONS USED FOR ANXIETY AND SLEEP DISTURBANCES

Objectives

The information in this chapter will assist you to:

» Identify the clinical features of a range of anxiety and sleep disturbances
» Describe the pathophysiology of anxiety and sleep disturbances
» Outline the pharmacology of anti-anxiety and hypnotic medications used to manage anxiety and sleep disturbances
» Understand consumer perspectives and experiences of having anxiety and sleep disturbances
» Outline prescribing and administration issues for anti-anxiety and hypnotic medications used to manage sleep disturbances

Key terms and abbreviations

Agoraphobia
Anxiety
Hypersomnia
Hypnotics
Insomnia
Parasomnia

CBT – cognitive behavioural therapy
GABA – gamma-aminobutyric acid
SNRIs – selective noradrenaline
   reuptake inhibitors
SSRIs – selective serotonin reuptake
   inhibitors

INTRODUCTION

In this chapter, we provide an overview of the pharmacological management of anxiety and sleep disturbances. As previously identified, while pharmacological agents are often significant and/or first-line treatments for most mental health problems, they exist within a clinical context that includes a range of treatment approaches, many of which are non-pharmacological. This is particularly true for these most common of problems – those of anxiety and sleep.

In the treatment and management of anxiety, psychotherapy (particularly cognitive behavioural therapy (CBT)), combined with antidepressant medications (particularly the selective serotonin reuptake inhibitors (SSRIs) and selective noradrenaline reuptake inhibitors (SNRIs)), are first-line options. Benzodiazepines and beta blockers are also used for time-limited anxiety problems or short-term management (Ohaeri 2006, Saeed et al 2007). See Table 5.1 for an overview of cognitive behavioural therapy. Many consumers find the combination of psychotherapeutic and pharmacological approaches to their anxiety helpful, and some find the option of psychotherapy alone to be more effective for managing their problem than the use of long-term medication.

TABLE 5.1 – COGNITIVE BEHAVIOURAL THERAPY (CBT)	
What CBT is	A commonly used psychotherapeutic approach that, as its name implies, focuses on a person's cognition (thoughts) and behaviour (actions). It works to alter thought processes in order to produce desired changes in their feelings and behaviours The emphasis in CBT is on challenging faulty assumptions and beliefs that the person has developed and teaching them coping skills that may be helpful in addressing their problems. It is a goal-directed and problem-focused therapy that focuses on present rather than past issues
What CBT is used for	Is often the treatment of choice for a range of mental health problems and has been used for managing depression, anxiety, schizophrenia, personality problems, eating disorders and bipolar disorder. It has also been found useful for insomnia, substance dependence and crisis intervention, and is used alone or in combination with medication, as either an individual or group therapy
Main features of CBT	CBT uses a range of structured cognitive techniques including questioning and challenging of assumptions and use of a diary to record events and associated thoughts, feelings and behaviours. Behavioural techniques include relaxation techniques and graded exposure

The combination of CBT and pharmacotherapy is also the most common approach to the treatment and management of sleep disturbances (Krystal et al 2006, Suhl 2007). Attention to lifestyle and daily habits is important for both anxiety and sleep disturbances. Effective overall management of both groups of disturbances therefore involves comprehensive attention to adequate diet and exercise, reduction of caffeine and alcohol intake, adequate sleep and stress reduction and management, as well as psychotherapeutic and pharmacological options. This chapter provides an overview of pharmacotherapy for anxiety disturbances and outlines sleep disturbances with a focus on the pharmacological management of insomnia.

ANXIETY

Anxiety disorders are associated with a person's perception of the threat of harm to other people or themselves, in which ambiguous stimuli may be misconstrued or distorted. This produces emotional, behavioural and motor responses that can be severe and debilitating. These responses include autonomic nervous system activation, changes in muscle tone, ritualised behaviours, sleep disturbances and alterations in attention and concentration.

Anxiety disorders are considered the most common types of mental health problem with a reported incidence in the USA of 18% (Kessler et al 2005a, 2005b). The prevalence of anxiety disorders in Australia is reported at 12 women per 100 000 and 7 men per 100 000 of the population (AIHW 2006), with most developing during childhood and adolescence or young adulthood. Unfortunately, there is a significant problem with under-diagnosis and therefore under-treatment of this group of disorders (Nash & Nutt 2007). This may be due, in part, to a perception by the general public that symptoms of anxiety are 'normal' or to be expected and tolerated so that they do not seek help for them. However, while they have sometimes been considered to be milder or less severe than other mental health problems, particularly those of psychotic depth, anxiety disturbances are often chronic mental health problems associated with significant personal distress and difficulty in managing daily functioning.

Anxiety disturbances have been associated with higher risk of suicide and substance abuse/dependence, poorer physical health, difficulties with sleep and problems with marital/relationship functioning (Ohaeri 2006). As noted in Chapter 4, they are also significantly co-morbid with depression. There are a number of forms of anxiety disturbance including panic attacks, social anxiety disorders, post-traumatic stress disorder, specific phobias, obsessive–compulsive disorder (OCD) and generalised anxiety disorder (see Chat box 5.1). While they produce a similar profile of responses, the triggers and duration of symptoms can vary greatly. Currently, there is some debate about whether OCD belongs to the group of anxiety disturbances. Pollack et al (2007) report that it may be better understood as belonging to a group of obsessive–compulsive spectrum disorders that are being considered as a separate diagnostic category in the forthcoming fifth edition of the Diagnostic and Statistical Manual of Mental Disorders (i.e. DSM V). The major characteristics of anxiety disturbances are summarised in Table 5.2.

PATHOPHYSIOLOGY OF ANXIETY DISTURBANCES

Human and animal studies investigating the neurobiology of fear, anxiety and aggression have shown that the amygdala is a key brain centre involved in the processing and expression of these emotions. The amygdalae are located bilaterally in the medial temporal lobes. The amygdala is also involved in emotional memory and the recognition of emotional states in other people. When the amygdalae are damaged, the

CHAT BOX 5.1 – LIVING WITH ANXIETY

A 28-year-old woman, working as an engineer, describes her experience of living with generalised anxiety that was diagnosed when she was 24:

By the time I was given the diagnosis, I was not surprised or upset because it had become quite clear to me that I had a problem. I was coping moderately well with life when a death in the family created extra stress. While I didn't feel any more depressed than seemed appropriate, I developed new symptoms, like chest pains. I became concerned that I may have developed a heart condition.

It is a big pain to live with anxiety disorder. I recently stopped taking medication, hoping that my calm feelings would continue, but that hasn't been the case. No matter how much I try to avoid it I find that my life is inhibited by my desire to avoid things that scare me.

I don't like trains, airplanes, subways, tunnels, high places, and low places. When I go to the movies I worry about being trapped in a fire so I try to sit near the aisle ...

I've always been a nervous person – even as a child – so I've learned to make light of my fears, but there are times when I can't control it. It can be very embarrassing.

(Adapted from Anonymous 2003, p 702)

TABLE 5.2 – CATEGORIES OF COMMON ANXIETY DISORDERS

Anxiety Disorder	Clinical features
Panic disorder	Sudden, spontaneous short-lived episode of intense anxiety
Agoraphobia	Feelings of anxiety in situations where escape or help may be difficult (e.g. outside the home, on public transport, in crowded public places)
Specific phobia	Fear or avoidance of specific situations or objects (e.g. fear of spiders, flying or needles)
Social phobia	Specific phobia associated with social situations that involve meeting new people, public performance or eating in public
Obsessive–compulsive disorder (OCD)	Unreasonable thoughts and fears experienced when engaging in recurrent, ritualised, seemingly purposeless behaviours to reduce the anxiety
Post-traumatic stress disorder (PTSD)	Anxiety following exposure to an extreme, traumatic or catastrophic event
Generalised anxiety disorder	Anxiety not associated with a specific event, object or situation

(Adapted from *Anxiety disorders and panic states, eMIMS 2007*, by J S Olver and G D Burrows 2006, CMPMedica Australia) affected person experiences a flattened affective state.

It has been proposed that the processing of fear and anxiety involves two pathways: the short loop or 'low road' and the long loop or 'high road' (Ohman 2005, LeDoux 1996). The short loop generates responses instantaneously to a stimulus, such as freezing and autonomic activation, that place the body on alert. Information is received by the thalamus and transferred to the amygdala, which in turn activates the hypothalamus and brain stem to initiate the visceral and behavioural responses. The long loop involves more conscious processing of the information, and considered decisions are made as to the nature of the stimulus and the appropriate level of responsiveness to follow. In this pathway there is interplay between the amygdala and cortical regions (prefrontal area, sensory cortex and insula) in the processing of the information (see Fig 5.1).

The caudate nucleus of the basal ganglia is also implicated in anxiety

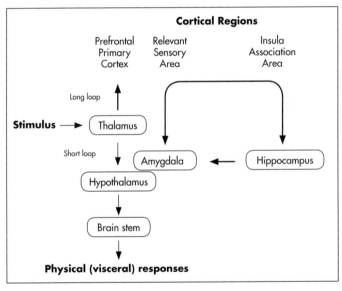

Figure 5.1 – The short and long loops involved in the processing of anxiety
In the short loop involved in processing anxiety, the stimulus is received by the thalamus and is transmitted to the amygdala. The amygdala initiates the physical responses associated with anxiety, producing an immediate and automatic reaction. In the long loop, the information is relayed, depending on the sensory mode, to the relevant areas of the cortex where characteristic features of the stimulus are consciously recognised and compared to past experience. Decisions are made as to the appropriate response and are relayed through the amygdala. The context of the stimulus is also processed by the hippocampus.
With permission from http//www.thebrain.mcgill.ca

states, particularly OCD. The caudate nucleus plays a role in automatic checking behaviours associated with familiar procedural tasks. These checking behaviours are part of well-learned procedures that usually happen below the level of conscious awareness and are aimed at minimising harm or threat. Examples are turning off the stove after cooking and locking a door as you are leaving your home. It has been proposed that in OCD, this implicit process becomes explicit. In other words, checking behaviours become conscious and deliberate acts. The current model of OCD pathophysiology (Neel et al 2002) suggests that two reinforced loops become established in the brains of affected persons (see Fig 5.2). The prefrontal cortex perceives a threat and consciously activates the caudate to initiate checking behaviours. This information passes back through the thalamus to the prefrontal cortex, but the perceived threat is not yet extinguished. The loop is activated again – resulting in compulsive, ritualised checking. The prefrontal cortex also activates the amygdala, resulting in an enhanced anxiety state. This feeds back through the thalamus to the prefrontal cortex, which can then further activate the amygdala. There is clearly interplay between these two loops as there is overlap between the brain regions involved. Neuroimaging studies have shown that the prefrontal areas of people affected with OCD show a larger volume than those without the disorder. It has been suggested that the larger regional volume may be due to poor 'pruning' of redundant neuronal connections early in development that predisposes these individuals to the establishment of such loops (Neel et al 2002, Rosenberg & Keshavan 1998).

Alterations in serotonergic, adrenergic and gamma-aminobutyric acid (GABAergic) neurotransmission have been implicated in anxiety disorders. There is evidence, particularly pharmacological, that an enhancement of these transmitter systems can be therapeutic in certain anxiety disorders. However, excessive stimulation of serotonergic and adrenergic systems in the brain can also induce anxiety states.

PHARMACOLOGY OF ANTI-ANXIETY MEDICATIONS

The pharmacological treatment of anxiety disorders comprises primarily the benzodiazepines and antidepressants and may include the non-benzodiazepine buspirone. Atypical antipsychotic medications such as risperidone and olanzapine and anti-seizure medications such as gabapentin are considered useful additional treatments for some anxiety disturbances, particularly those that have been treatment-resistant (Pollack et al 2007).

The choice of agent has less to do with the efficacy of anxiolytic action and more to do with the range and severity of adverse effects, the need for early onset of action and the co-existence of symptoms of depression

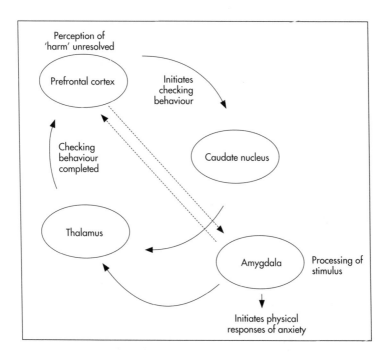

Figure 5.2 – Model of the circuitry involved in obsessive–compulsive disorder

(Tyrer & Baldwin 2006). The preferred anti-anxiety agents are now the antidepressant drugs; in particular, the SSRIs and NSRIs are considered first-line treatments for all major anxiety disturbances (Nash & Nutt 2007). Common antidepressant groups used include the SSRIs, the NSRI venlafaxine and the tetracyclic antidepressant mirtazapine. Older antidepressants such as the tricyclic antidepressants and the monoamine oxidase inhibitors have been shown to be effective in panic disorders; however, their use is limited because of the severity of their adverse effect profile. The mechanisms of action and common adverse effects of the antidepressants are described in Chapter 4.

Benzodiazepines are effective in relieving the symptoms of anxiety and also have sedative/hypnotic effects – i.e. they are sedating and calming and can induce sleep. In addition, they have anti-seizure, muscle relaxant and memory-impairing effects. Injectable forms of benzodiazepines such as midazolam are particularly effective in sedation and the management of agitation and behavioural emergencies associated with acute disturbances such as delirium and acute psychotic states (Therapeutic Guidelines 2003). Further details on the management of behavioural emergencies are given in Chapter 8.

The use of the benzodiazepines, such as alprazolam, diazepam and oxazepam, as anti-anxiety agents is now restricted to the acute treatment of anxiety disorders. See Table 5.3 for an overview of the benzodiazepines. While the onset of action of these drugs is relatively rapid (a tremendous advantage during the latent period before the full clinical benefits of the antidepressants develop, which can be 2–4 weeks), the adverse effects of treatment are considerable. Common adverse effects include drowsiness, light-headedness, dizziness, impaired motor coordination, visual disturbances, slurring of speech, lethargy, impaired memory, paradoxical agitation and poor concentration. The medications may have to be administered in high doses, making adverse effects more likely. While dependence on benzodiazepines is rare in consumers taking therapeutic doses for short periods such as 1–2 weeks, physical and psychological dependence can develop with longer term use, as can drug tolerance. Overdose may also be an issue, particularly when benzodiazepine use is combined with that of other sedatives. Sudden withdrawal of treatment with a benzodiazepine can initiate a withdrawal syndrome that can be severe. See Clinical alert box 5.1 for benzodiazepines.

TABLE 5.3 – BENZODIAZEPINES

Generic name	Australian trade names	New Zealand trade names	Daily dose range
Alprazolam	Xanax	Xanax	0.5–4 mg
Clonazepam	Rivotril	Rivotril	2–8 mg
Diazepam	Valium	D-Pam, Propam, Diazemuls, Stesolid Rectal	5–30 mg
Flunitrazepam	Rohypnol		0.5–2 mg
Lorazepam	Ativan	Ativan, Lorapam, Lorzem	2–4 mg
Nitrazepam	Mogadon	Insoma, Nitrados	5–10 mg
Oxazepam	Serepax	Ox-Pam, Serepax, Benzotran	45–90 mg
Temazepam	Normison	Normison, Somapam, Euhypnos	5–20 mg

(Therapeutic Guidelines 2003, New Zealand Medicines and Medical Devices Safety Authority 2008)

CLINICAL ALERT 5.1 – BENZODIAZEPINES: DEPENDENCE AND WITHDRAWAL

Physical and psychological dependence can develop with longer term use (i.e. weeks–months) of benzodiazepines, as can drug tolerance. Clients with a history of substance dependence are more likely to become dependent or misuse benzodiazepines. Thorough assessment of the risk/benefit ratio and use of concomitant substances is needed before prescribing these medications.

Sudden withdrawal of long-term treatment with a benzodiazepine can initiate a withdrawal syndrome that can be severe. When discontinuing treatment, the medication needs to be slowly withdrawn over a period of weeks–months.

Benzodiazepines act on the $GABA_A$ receptor complex within the CNS. They bind to the receptor and enhance the action of GABA when it interacts with the receptor. GABA has a key inhibitory influence on nerve pathways; it hyperpolarises the nerve membrane, making depolarisation and action potential generation less likely (see Fig 5.3). The $GABA_A$ receptor complex has a number of subunits associated with its structure. It has been reported that benzodiazepines that bind more selectively to the α_2 subunit of the complex can induce more specific anxiolytic actions, with fewer amnestic and sedative effects.

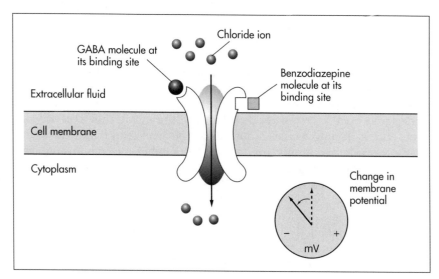

Figure 5.3 – The cellular mechanism of action of the benzodiazepines.
The benzodiazepines attach to a binding site on the GABA receptor, enhancing the action of GABA. This results in an influx of chloride ions and hyperpolarisation of the cell membrane, which inhibits impulse transmission.
From Fundamentals of Pharmacology (5th edn), 2007, by S Bullock, E Manias and A Galbraith, Prentice Hall, Fig 35.2, p 372, *with permission*

The non-benzodiazepine, buspirone, has a place in the management of anxiety disorders, especially generalised anxiety disorder. It acts as a partial agonist at serotonergic and dopaminergic receptors in the brain. Its advantages over the benzodiazepines are that the incidence of dependence and sedation is very low and that it can be used as long-term treatment. However, its disadvantage is that the onset of therapeutic benefit is delayed for a couple of weeks. Common adverse effects include tachycardia, visual disturbances and gastrointestinal upset.

Beta blockers can be useful in the acute management of the symptoms of anxiety during performance such as palpitations, sweating and tremor. Common adverse effects of beta blockers can be serious and include bradycardia and hypotension.

CONSUMER PERSPECTIVES ON ANXIETY AND ITS TREATMENT

For such a common group of mental health problems, there is comparatively little in the way of investigation of the lived experience of anxiety. While there are some individual accounts of the experience of having anxiety and co-morbid problems such as depression, there are few studies that have sought to describe what it is like to live with such a chronic and potentially debilitating condition.

Given its significant co-morbidity with depression and substance abuse, it is not surprising that descriptions of the experience of anxiety are often linked with depression. In a study by Haslam et al (2004), many of the 74 participants with anxiety and depression, some of whom were nurses and doctors, reported they had been unaware they had anxiety and depression until a crisis occurred in their lives, and that it was more often others such as family, friends and work colleagues who recognised the signs before they did. Physical symptoms of their illness were most identifiable to the participants, and these included dizziness, headaches, nausea and lack of energy. These often combined with other symptoms including tiredness, difficulty concentrating, having extremes of emotion and difficulty making decisions. Problems with sleep were common, and this often led to tiredness at work and the use of alcohol in an effort to self-medicate. As one participant describes:

> I started having one drink, then another at night – to knock me out so that I could sleep but even then I'd wake up at three o'clock in the morning with my mind racing – and then crawling to work, not hung over but just exhausted.
>
> (Haslam et al 2004, p 207)

According to these participants, the side effects of medication (which included SSRIs, other antidepressants and benzodiazepines) were similar to those of their anxiety and depression and included feeling dizzy, confused and nauseous and having difficulty making decisions. Not surprisingly, the side effects and/or the lack of improvement in their symptoms while taking the medications led to many participants non-adhering to them (Haslam et al 2004). One young woman explains that her medication made her feel worse than before:

> I found that really hard, because I felt so awful ... the tablets give you some nasty side effects of nausea ... it seems crazy that a tablet that's meant to help with those symptoms actually can make it worse to start with.
>
> (Haslam et al 2004, p 209)

Other participants, who had found their medications helpful, were still concerned that they might become dependent on them, and worried about how they would cope when they stopped taking them. Similarly to other studies of consumer perspectives on psychotropic medications, these participants found that health professionals who provided written and verbal information about their illness, medication and side effects, and took time to listen to their concerns, were the most helpful (see Comment box below). Self-help groups were also considered useful and, once again, GPs were identified as being one of the front-line health professionals in the diagnosis and treatment of their anxiety and depression (Haslam et al 2004).

COMMENT BOX – MANAGING PANIC DISORDER FROM A CONSUMER'S PERSPECTIVE

How could health professionals be more helpful?

Telling the person that they have panic disorder is not enough. You need to describe the symptoms to the person. They will be greatly relieved that their symptoms are being recognised. Providing an information leaflet, which includes a list of typical symptoms, can also be helpful.

The person should be reassured that there is a very successful treatment, but it requires their co-operation. There is no magic pill. If the patient is referred, it is important that they are seen by someone skilled in cognitive behaviour therapy.

(Adapted from McDonald 2000)

PRESCRIBING AND ADMINISTRATION ISSUES FOR ANTI-ANXIETY MEDICATIONS

- Prior to prescribing medication for anxiety, attention needs to be given to thorough history taking and physical and psychosocial assessment, including identification of co-morbid disorders (particularly alcohol/ substance misuse/dependence and depression).

- Assessment needs to include the impact of the anxiety disturbance on the consumer's occupation and social and/or domestic functioning.
- Use of screening tools for the disorder may be helpful in the assessment phase prior to prescribing. See Table 5.4 for a list of appropriate tools.
- Consumers need to be given adequate written and verbal information and education regarding the uses and potential side effects of anti-anxiety medications prior to prescription and administration.
- Benzodiazepines (particulary midazolam and lorazepam) are the medications of choice for sedation and should be given orally where possible (see Clinical alert 5.2).
- When considering benzodiazepines for anxiety, thorough assessment of the risk/benefit ratio and the use of concomitant substances is needed before prescribing these medications.

TABLE 5.4 – SCREENING AND OUTCOME MEASUREMENT TOOLS FOR ANXIETY	
Hamilton Anxiety Scale (HAMA)	A 14-item test measuring the severity of anxiety symptoms. It is also sometimes called the Hamilton Anxiety Rating Scale (HARS). A copy of the scale is available at: http://www.anxietyhelp.org/information/hama.html
Kessler Psychological Distress Scale (K10)	A 10-item self-report measure of psychological distress. A copy of the scale is available at: http://www.nevdgp.org.au/files/programsupport/mentalhealth/K10_English%5B1%5D.pdf?PHPSESSID=fc2ab9736eff3c44f9a0a2e27a3ab606
Hospital Anxiety and Depression Scale (HADS)	A 14-item self-report measure of depression and anxiety. Seven questions measure depression, and seven measure anxiety. A copy of the scale is available on payment at: http://www.onestopeducation.co.uk/icat/hospitalanxietyanddepress

CLINICAL ALERT 5.2 – INTRAMUSCULAR AND INTRAVENOUS BENZODIAZEPINE ADMINISTRATION
» Due to its poor and erratic absorption from muscle tissue, diazepam should not be given intramuscularly » Due to the risk of respiratory depression, midazolam should not be given intravenously

DISTURBANCES OF SLEEP

Disturbances of sleep may be grouped under the three broad headings of insomnia, hypersomnia and parasomnia. See Table 5.5 for an overview of the main types of sleep disturbances. Sleep disturbances are generally considered to be either primary sleep disturbances, which occur in isolation, or secondary sleep disturbances, which occur in association with either physical or mental health problems (Szabadi 2006).

TABLE 5.5 – TYPES OF SLEEP DISTURBANCES	
Sleep disturbance	Main features
Insomnia	An impairment in the quality of sleep in which the person has difficulty initiating or maintaining sleep and where the lack of sleep results in daytime fatigue, irritability, difficulty concentrating or other problems in functioning
Hypersomnia	Excessive daytime sleepiness (EDS) or prolonged night-time sleep. Causative/contributing factors include substance abuse, central nervous system injury, depression, epilepsy, obesity or other sleep disorders such as narcolepsy (i.e. EDS, cataplexy, disruption to night-time sleep pattern, hypnogogic hallucinations and sleep paralysis)
Parasomnia	Behavioural disturbances related to sleep, including sleepwalking, restless legs syndrome, teeth grinding and night terrors, which are often associated with stress and depression

Sleep disturbances are commonly linked with mental health problems, and these are one of the major causes of chronic insomnia in this client group, contributing to approximately 50% of cases. Indeed, the relationship between sleep and mental health problems can be considered to be synergistic, where one impacts upon the other. Hypersomnia, daytime sleepiness and fatigue are also common issues for these clients and, along with insomnia, can lead to a decline in clients' cognitive functioning, diminished productivity and an overall lower quality of life (Singh et al 2006).

INSOMNIA

Insomnia is one of the most common of the sleep disorders and is characterised by a difficulty in either getting to sleep or staying asleep. It may also be known by the rather cumbersome title disorders of initiating and maintaining sleep (DIMS). Insomnia usually suggests an underlying medical condition. It may also occur as a result of an adverse drug effect or as a part of the ageing process. Insomnia can be managed by behaviour modification, through better management of the existing medical condition or by the use of medicines that promote sleep. These agents are called hypnotics.

The benzodiazepines are a popular choice among prescribers for the short-term management of insomnia because they have good efficacy as hypnotics, a rapid onset and a mild adverse effect profile. The stages of sleep are outlined in Table 5.6. The benzodiazepines facilitate stage 2 sleep but suppress stages 3 and 4 as well as rapid eye movement (REM) sleep. The clinical consequences of these actions are to decrease the time taken to fall asleep and decrease awakenings during sleep. The choice of agent is dependent on whether the affected person has trouble getting to sleep or cannot remain asleep. Short-acting agents such as oxazepam and triazolam or the intermediate-acting temazepam are recommended in the former instance, whereas longer acting agents like nitrazepam, flunitrazepam and diazepam are more suitable in the latter. Morning or daytime drowsiness and impaired motor coordination can be problematic when the longer acting agents are used. After cessation of treatment a rebound in REM sleep may lead the person to experience vivid or nightmarish dreaming.

TABLE 5.6 – THE STAGES OF SLEEP

Stage	Features
REM sleep	Rapid eye movements, dreaming, increased or irregular heart and respiration rates, inhibition of skeletal muscles, increased cerebral activity, possible penile erection in men
Stage 1 non-REM sleep	Light sleep, reduced brain activity, slow eye movements and theta waves that characterise the electroencephalogram
Stage 2 non-REM sleep	Relaxed muscles, decreased body temperature, blood pressure and heart rate and sleep spindles that dominate the electroencephalogram
Stages 3 and 4 non-REM sleep	Deep sleep, bed-wetting/sleepwalking and delta waves that dominate the electroencephalogram

The elderly are particularly prone to insomnia due to age-related changes in sleeping patterns or increased use of medicines as a result of chronic illness. Benzodiazepine use can be problematic in the elderly. Changes in hepatic and renal function as a consequence of ageing or disease lead to an alteration in drug pharmacokinetics. Altered drug pharmacokinetics can lead to prolonged and/or increased drug effects. The elderly are also more sensitive to the effects of these drugs at the receptor level. This makes them more susceptible to the adverse effects of these drugs. It is therefore important to commence treatment for this group at lower doses than those given to younger adults.

The non-benzodiazepine hypnotics, zopiclone and zolpidem, are useful alternatives to the benzodiazepines. They are short-acting agents that do not interfere with REM sleep and produce less daytime sedation and impaired psychomotor function, but they still have the potential to induce dependence. See Medication in profile for zolpidem, which is commonly prescribed for insomnia.

MEDICATION IN PROFILE – ZOLPIDEM
Drug class: Non-benzodiazepine hypnotic
Uses and action: Used for the short-term treatment of insomnia where there is difficulty initiating sleep Effect appears to be due to its interaction with neuronal receptors that increase the inhibitory effect of GABA on neurones; similar sedative property to benzodiazepines
Daily dose range: 5–10 mg nocte (at bedtime)
Adverse effects: Diarrhoea, dizziness Paradoxical reactions can occur – e.g. hallucinations, agitation and rage – the medication needs to be discontinued in this circumstance Associated with potentially dangerous sleep-related behaviours such as sleep-walking and sleep-driving
Drug interactions and/or precautions: Caution is needed with clients who have hepatic insufficiency and with concomitant use of antidepressants Should not be used with alcohol Use should be limited to 4 weeks maximum under medical supervision

(*Therapeutic Guidelines* 2003, Therapeutic Goods Administration 2008)

Antidepressants with sedative action, such as the tricyclics and the tetracyclic mianserin, can also be useful in the management of depression with insomnia. However, elderly people are very sensitive to the antimuscarinic side effects of the tricyclics; reactions such as tachycardia, constipation, urinary retention, confusion and cognitive impairment can be problematic.

The sedating antihistamines, such as promethazine, trimeprazine and diphenhydramine, can be used as hypnotics in children and young people. Common adverse effects include daytime sedation and impaired performance and coordination, as well as dizziness. They can trigger paradoxical stimulation (especially in children), resulting in agitation, anxiety and hallucinations. They also tend to induce confusion and prolonged sleepiness when used in the elderly for this purpose and are not really recommended for this group of patients.

PRESCRIBING AND ADMINISTRATION ISSUES FOR MEDICATIONS USED TO TREAT INSOMNIA

- Prior to any pharmacological management, a thorough assessment and sleep history are needed. Assessment needs to focus on physical conditions and/or mental health problems that may be causative or co-morbid. History of substance use and current medications is also important, including the intake of alcohol, caffeine, nicotine and stimulants.
- Due to their potential for dependence, hypnotics should not be first-line treatment for insomnia. If prescribed, their use should be restricted to short-term and of limited duration.
- Use of long-term pharmacotherapy for the treatment of insomnia needs to be considered according to a number of factors. See Figure 5.4 for the steps to determine pharmacological appropriateness of treatment.

Conduct a thorough assessment of the client, including taking a comprehensive history and conducting a physical assessment

Assess the degree of functional impairment from the insomnia

Assess the risk/benefit ratio of other available treatment and management options

Contrast these with the risk/benefit ratio of pharmacotherapy based on available information

Assess the potential for abuse of the medication (those clients with substance abuse/dependence history or needing high dosages are considered the highest risks)

Figure 5.4 – Steps to determine long-term pharmacotherapy for chronic insomnia.
Adapted from Krystal et al 2006

CONCLUSIONS

This chapter has explored medications used to manage anxiety and sleep disturbances. These two major conditions are often, although not necessarily, linked. Psychotropic medications play a significant, although not exclusive, role in treating and managing both anxiety and sleep problems. It is important that clinicians understand the pathophysiology and pharmacology of anxiety and the related condition of depression, as well as that of sleep disturbances. Non-pharmacological treatments are often used concomitantly or instead of medication for these conditions. Regular and comprehensive assessment of consumers and carers is needed so that effective interventions can be used to reduce symptoms, manage side effects and enhance the wellbeing and quality of life of the person taking the medications, and of the family/carers who support them.

Useful websites

PADA – Panic Anxiety Disorder Association Inc, providing information and support for consumers, http://www.panicanxietydisorder.org.au

CRUfAD – Clinical Research Unit for Anxiety and Depression, providing resources, research and other information on anxiety and depression for consumers and clinicians, http://www.crufad.com/cru_index.html

The Phobic Trust – a New Zealand website promoting awareness and providing information and education on anxiety and related disorders, http://www.phobic.org.nz/

Recommended reading

Krystal A D, Rogers S, Fitzgerald M A 2006 Long-term pharmacotherapy in the management of chronic insomnia. The Journal for Nurse Practitioners 2(9):S621–S632

Nash J, Nutt D 2007 Psychopharmacology of anxiety. Psychiatry 6(4):143–148

Royal Australian and New Zealand College of Psychiatry (RANZCP) 2003 Clinical Practice Guidelines for the Treatment of Panic Disorder and Agoraphobia – comprehensive overview of panic disorder and agoraphobia, including psychotropic medication use. Available: http://www.ranzcp.org/pdffiles/cpgs/Panic%20Disorder%20and%20Agoraphobia%20Clinician%20Full.pdf

Teaching and learning activities

- Choose one of the medications used to treat anxiety or sleep disturbances. Do an online search for information on the particular medication. Use peer-reviewed sources and/or government/pharmaceutical information only. Develop a one-page profile of the medication, similar to the one provided in this chapter. Present it to your class for discussion.

References

Anonymous 2003 Commentary: A patient's story of living with anxiety. British Medical Journal 326:702

Australian Institute of Health and Welfare 2006 Australia's Health. AIHW Cat No AUS 73. AIHW, Canberra

Haslam C, Brown S, Atkinson S et al 2004 Patients' experiences of medication for anxiety and depression: Effects on working life. Family Practice 21(2):204–212

Kessler R C, Chiu W T, Demler O et al 2005a Prevalence, severity, and comorbidity of 12-month DSM-IV disorders in the National Comorbidity Survey Replication. Archives of General Psychiatry 62:617–627

Kessler R C, Berglund P, Demler O et al 2005b Lifetime prevalence and age-of-onset distributions of DSM-IV disorders in the National Comorbidity Survey Replication. Archives of General Psychiatry 62:593–602

Krystal A D, Rogers S, Fitzgerald M A 2006 Long-term pharmacotherapy in the management of chronic insomnia. The Journal for Nurse Practitioners 2(9):S621–S632

LeDoux J E 1996 The Emotional Brain. Simon and Shuster, New York

McDonald G 2000 Treatment of panic disorder: a personal experience. Australian Prescriber 23(6):127–128

Nash J, Nutt D 2007 Psychopharmacology of anxiety. Psychiatry 6(4):143–148

Neel J L, Stevens V M, Stewart J E 2002 Obsessive-compulsive disorder: Identification, neurobiology, and treatment. JAOA 102:81–86

New Zealand Medicines and Medical Devices Safety Authority (Medsafe) (2008) Regulatory Issues: Benzodiazepines to be controlled drugs. Available: http://www.medsafe.govt.nz/Profs/RIss/benzodiazepines.asp 14 Mar 2008

Ohaeri J U 2006 The management of anxiety and depressive disorders: A review. International Journal of Mental Health and Addiction 4:103–118

Ohman A 2005 The role of the amygdala in human fear: Automatic detection of threat. Psychoneuroendocrinology 30:953–958

Pollack M H, Otto M W, Roy-Byrne P P et al 2007 Novel treatment approaches for refractory anxiety disorders. Depression and Anxiety 0:1–10

Rosenberg D R, Keshavan M S 1998 Towards a neurodevelopmental model of obsessive-compulsive disorder. Biological Psychiatry 43:623–640

Saeed S A, Bloch R M, Antonacci D J 2007 Herbal and dietary supplements for treatment of anxiety disorders. American Family Physician 76:549–556

Singh A, Ghazvini P, Robertson N et al 2006 Sleep disturbances in patients with psychiatric illnesses. Journal of Pharmacy Practice 19(6):369–378

Suhl J 2007 The neuropharmacology of sleep disorders: Better sleeping through chemistry? Journal of Pharmacy Practice 20(2):181–191

Szabadi E 2006 Drugs for sleep disorders: Mechanisms and therapeutic prospects. British Journal of Clinical Pharmacology 61(6):761–766

Therapeutic Goods Administration 2008 Zolpidem ('Stilnox') – updated information – February 2008. Available: http://www.tga.gov.au/alerts/ stilnox2.htm (Department of Health and Ageing) 13 Mar 2008

Therapeutic Guidelines 2003 Therapeutic Guidelines: Psychotropic (5th edn) Therapeutic Guidelines Limited, North Melbourne, Australia

Tyrer P, Baldwin D 2006 Generalised anxiety disorder. Lancet 368:2156

CHAPTER 6

MEDICATIONS USED FOR SUBSTANCE USE PROBLEMS

Objectives:

The information in this chapter will assist you to:

» Identify the clinical features of a range of substance use problems

» Describe the pathophysiology of substance misuse and dependence

» Outline the pharmacology of medications used to manage substance misuse and dependence

» Understand consumer and carers' perspectives on substance use problems

» Outline prescribing and administration issues for medications used to manage substance use problems

Key terms and abbreviations

Dependence (addiction)
Dual diagnosis
Harmful use
Hazardous use
Licit/illicit drugs

Misuse
Tolerance
Withdrawal
AA – Alcoholics Anonymous
NA – Narcotics Anonymous

INTRODUCTION

There is a confusing array of terms used in the literature to refer to the use of, misuse/abuse of and dependence/addiction to substances, with some terms used interchangeably. Abuse is an ambiguous term with wide-ranging meaning that often carries stigma and refers to both harmful and hazardous use of a substance. In this chapter we will be using the term misuse to refer to the intake of a substance that results in potential harm or hazard to a person's physical and/or psychological health. Similarly, addiction is an older term that often carries stigma. Addiction includes a compulsion to take a substance and the subsequent development of tolerance to the substance over time, with associated withdrawal symptoms if substance intake is abruptly stopped or reduced. In this text, the more current term of dependence will be used.

In many countries, a number of substances, illicit and legal, are used for recreational purposes. Common reasons why these substances are taken include to induce pleasure and euphoria, provide relaxation, relieve stress or escape the negative feelings associated with mental illness; they may be taken as part of lifestyle experimentation or to achieve acceptance within a peer group. As noted, use becomes misuse when repeated administration becomes problematic, increasing the chances of illness, job loss, arrest and failure in life roles. Prolonged misuse can lead to dependence, where persistent, compulsive and uncontrolled use continues in spite of these problems, leading to maladaptive and destructive behaviours (Hyman 2005, Adinoff 2004). Drug dependence can trigger a withdrawal syndrome, which is characterised by physical discomfort and drug craving, when the use of the substance decreases or stops. The link between misuse and dependence, however, is not necessarily clear. A person's substance misuse does not always progress to dependence, and research indicates that the intake of some substances that have the potential for dependence (e.g. cocaine, heroin) does not automatically lead from one state to the other (Ridenour et al 2003).

Commonly misused substances include tobacco (nicotine), alcohol, narcotics, amphetamines, cocaine, marijuana, ecstasy and related drugs, hallucinogens, benzodiazepines and inhalable solvents. As noted, these substances can be broadly grouped under two headings – licit (or legal) and illicit/illegal substances. In Australia, the most commonly misused legal substances include alcohol and tobacco. In 2004, the most commonly used illicit drug in Australia was cannabis, with 1 in 3 people (34%) having used it during their lifetime, and 11% of the population having used it during that year. Methamphetamine had also been used by 9% of Australians over the age of 14, with 3% having used it within that year (AIHW 2007). A summary of recent Australian and New Zealand statistics on drug use is provided in Table 6.1.

SUBSTANCE USE AND MENTAL HEALTH – DUAL DIAGNOSIS

With respect to mental health, substance use and misuse are important issues. Dual diagnosis, or co-morbidity, refers to the presence of both a substance use problem and a mental health problem. Prevalence rates for co-existing problems indicate that between 35% and 60% of people with mental health problems also have a substance use issue (Mueser et al. 1995 and Menezes et al 1996 in Rassool 2006). The links between substance misuse and mental health are complex, where one may be considered the 'primary' problem and the other 'secondary'. Often, however, it is difficult to determine which problem came first. What is important is that both the substance use problem and the mental health problem are addressed because, if only one is treated and not the other, the consumer is much less likely to recover from either issue.

TABLE 6.1 – RECENT REGIONAL STATISTICS ON SUBSTANCE USE

Substance	Features
Tobacco	• 17% Australians aged 14 years and over were daily smokers • In 1999, 26% of New Zealand adults were smokers • 26% Australians were ex-smokers • Men more likely to smoke than women, though in 1999 women aged 15–24 years in New Zealand had higher rates than men of the same age • Between 1991 and 2004, smoking rates declined in Australia and a similar trend was seen in New Zealand between 1989 and 1999
Alcohol	• In 2004, 84% Australians aged 14 years and over had consumed at least one alcoholic drink in the last 12 months • In 1995, 87% of New Zealanders aged 14–65 years had consumed at least one alcoholic drink in the last 12 months • 9% Australians consume alcohol on a daily basis • 41% Australians most likely to drink on a weekly basis • Australian males more likely to consume alcohol than women
Illicit drugs	• 28% Australians aged 14 and over had used an illicit drug at least once in their lifetime, 15% at least once in the last 12 months • Cannabis was the most commonly used illicit drug in Australia, 33% having used it at least once in their lifetime, 11% having used it in the last 12 months • Cannabis is the third most popular recreational drug in New Zealand after alcohol and tobacco • In 1998 the New Zealand National Drug Survey revealed that, in the 18–24 age group, 43% males and 27% females had used cannabis in the last 12 months • In 2004, illicit drug use in Australia was most prevalent in persons aged 18–29 years • In 2004, the proportion using ecstasy was 3% in Australia, the highest prevalence for this substance over the period 1991–2004 • In 2004, the most prevalent drugs in the ecstasy and related drug group used by 12–24-year-olds in Australia were ecstasy and methamphetamine/amphetamines

(Adapted from *Statistics on drug use in Australia 2004, 2005,* by the Australian Institute of Health and Welfare, AIHW Cat No PHE 62, AIHW [Drug Statistic Series No 15] and *New Zealand Drug Statistics,* 2001, by the New Zealand Health Information Service, New Zealand Ministry of Health)

Substance use that has been particularly linked with mental health includes that of cannabis, and this is especially so for young people. There is considerable evidence that frequent use of cannabis may be predictive of a higher risk of developing psychotic symptoms (Hall 2006). Regular (i.e. daily–weekly) cannabis use has also been linked closely with the development of mental health problems such as depression and bipolar disorder (van Laar et al 2007). Research has also revealed that consumers with psychotic mental health problems such as schizophrenia and bipolar disorder show a significantly higher lifetime prevalence of illicit substance use, particularly of stimulants such as amphetamine and cocaine, than the general population (Ringen et al 2008).

While the focus of discussion in this chapter will be on the pharmacological management of substance dependence and withdrawal states, it is important to keep in mind that pharmacological treatment will be used within the context of overall management of a consumer's substance use problem. This will often include medical treatment for any co-existing physical health problems, psychiatric treatment of any co-existing mental health problems, and counselling for social and psychological issues and effects relating to the substance use problem. Therapeutic interventions such as cognitive behavioural therapy and/or motivational interviewing, harm reduction strategies, relapse prevention strategies, detoxification, withdrawal and rehabilitation programs and/or referral to self-help groups such as Alcoholics Anonymous (AA) or Narcotics Anonymous (NA) are also effective options.

PATHOPHYSIOLOGY OF SUBSTANCE USE PROBLEMS

The medications used in the management of substance misuse are directed towards controlling the effects of dependence – drug cravings and the withdrawal syndrome. Studies of the neurobiology of drug seeking or dependent behaviour suggest that it is a dysfunction of the learning and the reward-reinforcement systems.

Normally humans, like other animals, develop goals that contribute to survival – such as seeking out food, shelter and mating – and these biological goals are seen as natural rewards. Cognitive and experiential rewards are associated with friendship and social status (Kalivas & Volkow 2005).

According to the model proposed by Hyman (2007), rewards are seen as desirable; they make us feel good and we are highly motivated to pursue them. Learned associations in our environment become cues to predict the availability of these rewards and they, in turn, trigger behaviours directed towards achieving these goals. Over time an increase in frequency in these behaviours reinforces the learning. Within the prefrontal cortex, there is a weighting of our goals according to their relative importance. With reinforcement, the actions required to obtain a reward become automatic and very efficient via connections to subcortical structures. Hyman states that behavioural control is the domain of the prefrontal cortex and its connections to the thalamus and corpus striatum and is achieved by maintaining the goal representation over time, suppressing distraction and inhibiting impulsiveness.

This circuitry is influenced by the activity of a dopaminergic modulatory system called the mesocorticolimbic pathway (see Fig 6.1). Dopamine is released from neurones in the ventral tegmental area (VTA) within the midbrain. These neurones project to a number of brain regions, in particular the amygdala, nucleus accumbens and prefrontal cortex, reinforcing a particular reward and altering the relative value of our other goals in relation to this one. An increase in dopaminergic activity signals that a reward is new or better than expected and this promotes learning. After repeated exposure the learned experience becomes very familiar and there is no increase in dopaminergic activity (Schultz et al 1997, Schultz 1998, 2006).

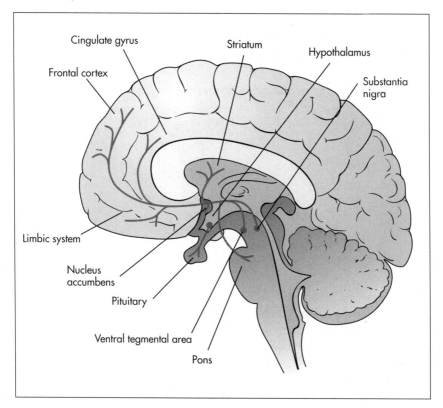

Figure 6.1 – The mesocorticolimbic pathway.
Reproduced from Pathophysiology (3rd edn), 2005, by L C Copstead and J L Banasik, Elsevier-Saunders, Fig 43.32A, p 1077, with permission

As dependence develops, this process becomes pathological. The drug repeatedly increases dopaminergic transmission, reinforcing that the reward is better than expected. This pathological learning alters the importance of all goals established within the prefrontal cortex relative to wanting the drug and reduces behavioural control (Hyman 2007). Some substances, such as cocaine and the amphetamines, alter synaptic dopamine concentrations in the nucleus accumbens directly. Other substances act indirectly to increase synaptic dopamine levels via G protein-coupled receptors or ligand-gated ion channel receptors (Adinoff 2004) (see Table 6.2). Several neurotransmitter systems have been implicated along with dopamine in the reinforcing effects of drug use, including endogenous opioids, GABA and the endocannabinoids. Furthermore, regional changes in the levels of GABA, glutamate, serotonin, dopamine and nicotine have been reported in association with withdrawal of abused substances (Koob 2006). The compulsion to take drugs may be associated with reciprocal glutamatergic projections from the prefrontal cortex and amygdala, as well as from the prefrontal cortex to the nucleus accumbens and VTA, forming a repeating loop within the mesocorticolimbical pathway (Adinoff 2004) (see Fig 6.1).

TABLE 6.2 – SUBSTANCES THAT INDIRECTLY INDUCE INCREASED MESOCORTICOLIMBIC DOPAMINE LEVELS	
Mechanism	Substance
G protein-coupled receptors	Tetrahydrocannabinol (THC) – active ingredient of cannabis Opioids Caffeine
Ion channel receptors	Alcohol Phencyclidine (PCP) – an hallucinogen Nicotine

(From Adinoff 2004)

There are a number of risk factors associated with substance misuse, including family history and gender (with males being at greater risk). Genetics also plays a role in determining the sensitivity of receptor systems, enzyme levels and metabolism that may contribute to a vulnerability to misuse substances. For example, there is evidence that the prevalence of particular genotypes associated with enzymes involved in alcohol metabolism within certain ethnic groups (for example, in South-East Asian people) may be protective against alcohol abuse and dependence (Moore et al 2007, Eng et al 2007).

An interesting area of research has developed to explore the basis of relapse, especially after an extended period of drug abstinence. It is proposed that dependence leads to long-lasting and stable remodelling of the brain circuits within the mesolimbic system. Two transcription factors, cAMP response element binding protein (CREB) and *deltaFosB*, that are responsible for the regulation of the expression of specific genes have become closely linked to chronic administration of addictive drugs because they can accumulate and persist in the prefrontal cortex and amygdala for an extended period (Nestler 2004). Nestler (2001) had already suggested that these factors may act as a switch that retains the connection between drug associated cues and reward long after drug use stops.

PHARMACOLOGICAL MANAGEMENT OF SUBSTANCE MISUSE

The management of substance misuse by medication can be classified as treatment of acute intoxication and the management of withdrawal syndromes associated with chronic misuse and dependence. The focus of this discussion will be on substances for which specific but limited pharmacotherapy is recommended as part of the management of substance withdrawal, specifically alcohol, opioids and nicotine (see Table 6.3).

TABLE 6.3 – SYMPTOMS OF COMMON SUBSTANCE WITHDRAWAL STATES

Type of withdrawal	Features of the withdrawal syndrome
Alcohol withdrawal (and other CNS depressants)	Tremor, disorientation, clouded consciousness, sweating, nausea and vomiting, visual and/or tactile hallucinations, paranoid delusions, anxiety and/or agitation, seizures; severe withdrawal may lead to delirium tremens (approximately 10% mortality) Onset usually 6–24 hours after the last drink, persisting for 72 hours and up to several weeks
Cannabis withdrawal (including marijuana, hashish)	Insomnia, hyperactivity, irritability, anxiety, depression, loss of appetite Onset can be as soon as 4 hours after cessation, peak between 4 and 7 days after and last for up to 2 weeks
Hallucinogen withdrawal (e.g. ecstasy, LSD, ketamine)	No clinical features
Sedative-hypnotic withdrawal (e.g. benzodiazepines, barbiturates)	Insomnia, anxiety, tremor, palpitations, sensory disturbances (e.g. hallucinations), seizures, possible death

TABLE 6.3 – SYMPTOMS OF COMMON SUBSTANCE WITHDRAWAL STATES cont'd	
Type of withdrawal	Features of the withdrawal syndrome
Opiates and opioids (e.g. heroin, methadone, morphine and codeine)	Runny nose, watering eyes, appetite loss, tremor, sweating, nausea, gooseflesh, diarrhoea, hypertension, panic, agitation, abdominal cramps, seizures Effects peak at 2–3 days and last for 5–7 days
Stimulants (e.g. amphetamines, cocaine, anabolic steroids)	Hypersomnia, irritability, aggression, depression, craving, anhedonia

(Adapted from Rassool & Winnington 2006, *Therapeutic Guidelines* 2003)

A major problem associated with the treatment of chronic substance misuse is that the rate of relapse can be very high. The reasons for this tend to centre on the physical and psychological dependence induced by these substances, access to effective management strategies and the demand on detoxification programs, as well as the nature of support systems from family and friends.

In acute intoxication, the management is directed towards preventing or attenuating symptoms such as dysrhythmias, infarction, aspiration, respiratory arrest, psychosis, alterations in blood pressure, seizures and hypoxic brain injury. General symptoms of intoxication are shown in Box 6.1. Examples of the treatments used to address these symptoms are summarised in Table 6.4.

There are specific antidotes available for the treatment of some forms of overdose: naloxone in the case of narcotic intoxication and flumazenil where benzodiazepine poisoning is determined. Naloxone is an opioid receptor antagonist that displaces the narcotic from the receptor and alleviates most of the symptoms of intoxication. Flumazenil is a benzodiazepine receptor antagonist that can lead to rapid reversal of intoxication with these drugs. Both of these antidotes are injected in acute situations and have shorter half-lives relative to the agents of intoxication, so the person being treated requires monitoring for signs of relapse into the overdosed state. Common adverse effects of flumazenil include agitation, nausea and vomiting. Flumazenil needs to be used with caution in chronic benzodiazepine users, as it can induce a rapid withdrawal syndrome that can trigger seizures and delirium.

ALCOHOL DEPENDENCE

The drugs used in the treatment of chronic alcohol dependence are directed towards reducing the withdrawal syndrome (acamprosate), reducing the

BOX 6.1 – SYMPTOMS OF INTOXICATION

Intoxication is an acute, temporary condition that follows the intake of alcohol or other psychoactive substance. Symptoms of intoxication lead to disturbances in a person's:
» level of consciousness
» cognition and perception
» affect and/or behaviour
» physical functioning.

The level of intoxication is dependent on the type of substance used, the dose, the person's tolerance to the substance and other factors including body weight, whether they have eaten prior to intake, over what time period the substance was taken and whether it was taken with other substances.

Intoxication symptoms depend on the particular effects the substance has on the central nervous system (e.g. CNS depressant, stimulant, sedative-hypnotic, hallucinogenic, etc.).

Common general symptoms of intoxication can include:
» feelings of euphoria
» uninhibited behaviour
» lack of motor coordination
» impaired judgment and decision making.

TABLE 6.4 – EXAMPLES OF TREATMENTS USED IN ACUTE SUBSTANCE INTOXICATION

Toxic effect of substance	Management
Excitation, confusion, anxiety	Sedation using a benzodiazepine
Psychosis	Antipsychotic agent
Dysrhythmias	Beta blocker
Opioid-induced respiratory depression and coma	Opioid antagonist, naloxone
Seizures	Anticonvulsant
Aspiration, hypoventilation, hypoxic brain injury, cardiovascular complications	Appropriate life support

cravings (naltrexone) and avoiding alcohol (disulfiram). These drugs are adjuncts to other management strategies that reduce alcohol consumption and maintain abstinence (Whelan 2002).

Acamprosate acts to decrease glutamatergic transmission in the brain by modulating NMDA glutamate receptor activity. Increased levels of glutamatergic transmission in the brain develop with chronic alcohol abuse. This heightened level of transmission that persists after cessation of alcohol abuse is thought to contribute, at least in part, to the withdrawal syndrome. Treatment is well tolerated, with headache, diarrhoea, pruritis and lowered libido being the most common adverse effects.

Like naloxone, naltrexone is an opioid receptor antagonist. Naltrexone has a longer half-life and is more effective orally than naloxone. It is believed to reduce cravings by inhibiting the activation of dopaminergic pathways involved in reward. Common adverse reactions include nausea, headache, dizziness, nervousness and fatigue. Liver function needs to be monitored during therapy.

Disulfiram has long been used to promote abstinence in people with chronic alcohol abuse problems by making them feel physically ill after ingestion of the substance. It inhibits an enzyme involved in the metabolism of alcohol called aldehyde dehydrogenase. This allows the metabolite, acetaldehyde, to accumulate in the body, which induces a variety of unpleasant symptoms. Acetaldehyde is a potent vasodilator, triggering flushing followed by a throbbing headache. Nausea, vomiting, sweating, respiratory difficulties, changes in blood pressure and feelings of unease are also commonly associated with this therapy. Rarely, hepatotoxicity and psychotic reactions can develop.

Benzodiazepine therapy with diazepam or oxazepam is also useful in the acute management of alcohol detoxification.

OPIOID WITHDRAWAL

An important treatment approach in opioid withdrawal has been to substitute the abused opioid with another opioid drug that can be better managed clinically. The main substitute opioid has been methadone, but there is increasing use of the partial agonist, buprenorphine, for this purpose (see Table 6.5). The rationale for the use of these opioids is that they have a much longer duration of action than other drugs from this class (24 hours for methadone and 6–8 hours for buprenorphine compared to 2–4 hours for the others), which leads to less craving and weaker withdrawal symptoms. Prolonged occupation of opioid receptors by these agents also means that the euphoric high is attenuated if the user administers another opioid because of the absence of available receptors to interact with it. Methadone can also be taken orally, reducing the risk of infection associated with self-injection and sharing of syringes. Buprenorphine can be taken as a sublingual preparation or applied as a transdermal patch. These formulations represent convenient, non-invasive forms of administration and require the user to attend a clinic on a regular basis for treatment and maintain therapeutic contact with health professionals. Another opioid agent that has been used in other countries in opioid substitution therapy is the partial agonist, L-acetyl methadol (LAAM). It has a longer half-life than methadone, so does not need to be administered as frequently. Unfortunately, it can cause cardiac dysrhythmias in some patients and is still not widely available in Australia.

TABLE 6.5 – TREATMENT OF LONG-TERM OPIOID DEPENDENCE		
Medication	**Effect**	**Suggested administration and dose**
Buprenorphine	Partial opioid agonist, effective in reducing illicit opioid use	Normally once daily 2–8 mg sublingually, initially over 2–3 weeks, then 8–24 mg maintenance, once daily or up to 32 mg on alternate days
Methadone	Synthetic opioid used as substitute for heroin and other opioids, effective in reducing their use	Dose will be dependent on amount of opioid used prior and initial response to methadone 20 mg orally daily, initially over 3 weeks, then doses above 50 mg daily = better outcome
Naltrexone	Long-acting pure opioid antagonist, effective in blocking effects of heroin	Naltrexone challenge test recommended prior to commencing, to confirm abstinence from opioids 25 mg orally as initial dose, then, if tolerated, increase next day to 50 mg daily

(Adapted from *Therapeutic Guidelines* 2003)

Naltrexone, used in the treatment of alcohol misuse, can also be used as an adjunct in the management of cravings in opioid withdrawal. As it is an opioid antagonist, withdrawal syndrome will occur after administration. A controversial form of naltrexone therapy, called rapid opiate detoxification, involves the administration of the drug while the person is sedated or anaesthetised over a number of days. The use of this approach means that the experience of the withdrawal syndrome is lessened. Proponents have claimed astonishing results, but these findings are disputed. Wodak (2001) reported that the treatment results are modest for street users, but are more successful as part of a comprehensive program or when used in highly 'motivated' patients.

Pharmacological relief of the symptoms of withdrawal, such as diarrhoea, muscle cramping, abdominal pain and insomnia, is also a standard part of opioid dependence management programs.

NICOTINE WITHDRAWAL

The damaging effects of cigarette smoking on health are well established. Smokers develop an addiction to the nicotine present in tobacco. The main pharmacological approach used in the management of nicotine withdrawal is to substitute the nicotine present in a cigarette with a pharmaceutical form of nicotine, free of other toxic contaminants present in cigarettes, and then to gradually wean the person off the substance. The cravings associated with the weaning off period are managed with antidepressant therapy using either bupropion or the tricyclic antidepressant nortryptyline.

Nicotine replacement therapy can be provided in the form of chewing gum, inhalants and transdermal patches. Common local adverse effects with the chewing gum and inhalants include sore or irritated throat, sore jaw, increased saliva production and bitter taste. The patch can cause local irritation and redness of the skin at the site of application. General side effects associated with the action of nicotine include headache, gastrointestinal discomfort, nausea and vomiting, dependence and palpitations.

The antidepressants are thought to act via the modulation of dopamine transmission in the brain associated with reward, most likely within the nucleus accumbens. The tricyclic antidepressants were covered in Chapter 3. The range of antimuscarinic and antiadrenergic adverse effects associated with this group need to be kept in mind when they are administered. Buproprion can cause headache, facial flushing, insomnia, tachycardia, hypertension, impaired concentration and anxiety. More rarely it can precipitate depression and suicidal ideation.

CONSUMER AND CARER PERSPECTIVES ON SUBSTANCE MISUSE

The social, occupational, physical, mental and emotional impacts of substance misuse and dependence can be significant and far-reaching. The misuse of alcohol, a socially accepted and readily available substance, is particularly high. As with most substance use, alcohol misuse often begins in late adolescence and young people often do not seek help for misuse and dependence until their situation is critical. Wells, Horwood and Fergusson (2007) report that, in a study where 351 young people aged 25 years were identified as having alcohol use problems, only 7% of participants had made any contact with alcohol and drug treatment services for their problems. Most of the young people reported they did not seek help because they thought they could handle the problem themselves, and some thought the problem would get better on its own. Some also did not think to seek help.

People who become dependent on substances report a number of reasons as to why they think they developed their problem. In one study exploring the experiences of men with alcohol dependence, the men reported they initially drank in order to manage feelings of insecurity, inadequacy and low self-esteem. Yet, paradoxically, seeking control over their feelings ended in an eventual loss of control over their drinking and other behaviours as they slid into dependency on the alcohol. This included awareness that their relationships with family and friends became compromised due to intoxicated behaviours (Zakrewski & Hector 2004). Indeed, the need to dampen down feelings, manage stress and/or to gain confidence to interact socially with others is a common thread in consumers' reports as to why they started using substances.

These findings also lend support to the fact that, often, it is other people in the person's life who first recognise the symptoms of their substance misuse, sometimes long before the person does. A number of studies have explored the experiences of family and friends who care for a person who is substance misusing and, as the onset of substance misuse often starts in adolescence, some have focused on this area. A recent Australian study by Usher, Jackson and O'Brien (2007), for instance, explored the experience of 18 parents whose children were misusing substances including alcohol, marijuana, amphetamines and ecstasy. Parents reported a number of issues, including: feeling guilt and shame about their child's drug use; having difficulty setting limits and dealing with the consequences of drug-related behaviours including verbal abuse, accidents and stealing; and grieving for the loss of the child they could have had but for the effects of the substance use. Guilt was a strong theme in their accounts:

> I thought … I had failed. I failed as a mum. Why did I not see this, why could I not protect my son from this? Why couldn't I make him better? … But until then it was where have I gone wrong? You speak to these other people and think, how did their son or daughter get into this?
>
> (Usher et al 2007, p 428)

Parents also discussed the issue of blame for their child's substance use problem and identified how they as parents were often blamed for the issue, when perhaps it could be better understood as a social problem:

> It is a problem society needs to deal with, but because they don't want to look at it, you just get blamed with the whole lot. I would not go to the police or the ambulance ever again. There's too much blame that goes on, um and me being his mother, I know that I cop a fair amount of that blame. Meanwhile the family just becomes more and more dysfunctional …
>
> (Usher et al 2007, p 426)

PRESCRIBING AND ADMINISTRATION ISSUES FOR MEDICATIONS USED FOR SUBSTANCE MISUSE

- Prior to prescribing and administration, taking a thorough history and making an assessment of physical and mental health and concomitant medications are necessary.
- Consumers need to be given adequate written and verbal information and education regarding the uses and potential side effects of medications such as naltrexone, methadone and buprenorphine prior to prescribing and administration.
- Caution is needed if prescribing benzodiazepines for the management of withdrawal, particularly for clients who are community-based, as these medications are commonly abused and, if combined with opioids such as heroin, may lead to overdose.
- When prescribing buprenorphine, caution is needed as it may precipitate a withdrawal state if used too closely to a high intake/ dose of an opioid.
- Education of and information for family/carers about medications and the potential for adverse effects and/or overdose, particularly for withdrawal programs in the community, are important.

CONCLUSIONS

This chapter has explored medications used to manage problems with substance use and dependence. Substance misuse is commonly co-morbid with mental health problems such as depression and psychosis. Psychotropic medications play an important, although not exclusive, role in treating and managing withdrawal and dependence. A comprehensive approach to addressing the psychosocial and physical effects of misuse and dependence is also needed to enhance the likelihood of successful outcomes. Clinicians need to understand the pathophysiology and pharmacology of substance use problems and be aware of the perspectives and needs of both consumers and family/carers. Comprehensive assessment of consumers and carers is needed so that effective interventions can be used to enhance the wellbeing and recovery of the person taking the medications and for the family/carers who support them.

Useful websites

Alcoholics Anonymous – providing information and support for people with alcohol dependence, as well as information on alcohol dependence for health professionals, http://www.alcoholics-anonymous.org/en_information_aa.cfm
Narcotics Anonymous – providing information and support for people with drug

dependence, as well as information on drug dependence for health professionals, http://www.na.org/

Drug Info Clearinghouse – national website and drug prevention network provided by the Australian Drug Foundation, has information about alcohol and other drugs and drug prevention, for consumers and professionals, http://www.druginfo.adf.org.au/

Recommended reading

Linford-Hughes A, Welch S 2006 Pharmacotherapeutic interventions in alcohol and illicit drug dependence. Psychiatry 6(1):5–11

Teaching and learning activities

• Using the information and quotes on carers' perspectives of having family members with substance use problems, discuss the following:

   a. How can issues of guilt, shame and blame impact on the person who is substance misusing and their family and friends? Is it a social issue we all need to take responsibility for? Are parents and others to blame for a person's substance misuse?

   b. How can family and friends of people who are substance misusing be supported by health professionals?

References

Adinoff B 2004 Neurobiologic processes in drug reward and addiction. Harvard Review of Psychiatry 12:305–320

Australian Institute of Health and Welfare (AIHW) 2007 Statistics on drug use in Australia 2006. Drug statistics series No 18. Cat. no. PHE 80. AIHW, Canberra

Eng M Y, Luczak S E, Wall T L 2007 ALDH2, ADH1B, and ADH1C genotypes in Asians: A literature review. Alcohol Res Health 30:22–27

Hall, W D 2006 Cannabis use and the mental health of young people. Australian and New Zealand Journal of Psychiatry 40:105–113

Hyman S E 2005 Addiction: a disease of learning and memory. American Journal of Psychiatry 162:1414–1422

Hyman S E 2007 The neurobiology of addiction: Implications for voluntary control of behaviour. American Journal of Bioethics 7:8–11

Kalivas P W, Volkow N D 2005 The neural basis of addiction: A pathology of motivation and choice. American Journal of Psychiatry 162:1403–1413

Koob G F 2006 The neurobiology of addiction: A neuroadaptational view relevant for diagnosis. Addiction 101(Suppl 1):23–30

Moore S, Montane-Jaime L K, Carr L G et al 2007 Variations in alcohol-metabolising enzymes in people of East Indian and African descent from Trinidad and Tobago. Alcohol Res Health 30:28–30

Nestler E J 2001 Molecular basis of long-term plasticity underlying addiction.

National Review of Neuroscience 2:119–128

Nestler E J 2004 Historical review: Molecular and cellular mechanisms of opiate and cocaine addiction. Trends in Pharmacological Science 25:210–218

Rassool G H 2006 Dual diagnosis nursing. Blackwell Publishing, Oxford

Rassool G H 2006 Understanding dual diagnosis: An overview. In: Rassool G H (ed) Dual diagnosis nursing. Blackwell Publishing, Oxford, pp 3–15

Rassool G H, Winnington J 2006 Dealing with intoxication, overdose, withdrawal and detoxification: Nursing assessment and interventions. In: Rassool G H (ed) Dual diagnosis nursing. Blackwell Publishing, Oxford, pp 186–195

Ridenour T A, Cottler L B, Compton W M et al 2003 Is there a progression from abuse disorders to dependence disorders? Addiction 98:635–644

Ringen P A, Melle I, Birkenaes A B et al 2008 Illicit drug use in patients with psychotic disorders compared with that in the general population: A cross-sectional study. Acta Psychiatrica Scandinavica 117(2):133–138

Schultz W 1998 Predictive reward signal of dopamine neurons. Journal of Neurophysiology 80:1–27

Schultz W 2006 Behavioral theories and the neurophysiology of reward. Annual Review of Psychology 57:87–115

Schultz W, Dayan P, Montague P R 1997 A neural substrate of prediction and reward. Science 275:1593–1599

Therapeutic Guidelines 2003 Therapeutic Guidelines: Psychotropic (5th edn) Therapeutic Guidelines Limited, North Melbourne, Australia

Usher K, Jackson D, O'Brien L 2007 Shattered dreams: Parental experiences of adolescent substance abuse. International Journal of Mental Health Nursing 16(6):422–430

van Laar M, van Dorsselaer S, Monshouwer K et al 2007 Does cannabis use predict the first incidence of mood and anxiety disorders in the adult population? Addiction 102:1251–1260

Wells J E, Horwood J, Fergusson D M 2007 Reasons why young adults do or do not seek help for alcohol problems. Australian and New Zealand Journal of Psychiatry 41(12):1005–1012

Whelan G 2002 The management of the heavy drinker in primary care. Australian Prescriber 20:70–73

Wodak A 2001 Drug treatment for opioid dependence. Australian Prescriber 24:4–6

Zakrzewski R F, Hector M A 2004 The lived experiences of alcohol addiction: Men of alcoholics anonymous. Issues in Mental Health Nursing 25:61–77

Unit 3
Special Issues

CHAPTER 7

ISSUES RELATED TO THE PRESCRIPTION AND USE OF PSYCHOTROPIC MEDICATION IN SPECIAL POPULATIONS

Objectives

The information in this chapter will assist you to:

» Outline the key issues related to the use of psychotropic medications in special populations

» Understand the main disorders for which psychotropic medications are prescribed for use with pregnant or breastfeeding women, children and adolescents and the older person

» Describe the clinical implications of using psychotropic medications with pregnant or breastfeeding women, children and adolescents, the elderly and Indigenous peoples

» Outline the serious adverse reactions that may occur with each of these groups of people and how they might be managed

» Understand the importance of considering the ethical perspective related to the use of these medications, especially with regard to their use in children and the older person

Key terms and abbreviations

'Floppy baby' syndrome
Immediate post-partum period
In-utero
Placenta
Placental transfer
Polypharmacy
Switching
Teratogenic effects
Therapeutic orphans
Tic disorders
Tourette's syndrome

ADD – attention deficit disorder
ADHD – attention deficit/ hyperactivity disorder
DLPFC – dorsolateral prefrontal cortex
DBDs – disruptive behavioural disorders
EPSE – extrapyramidal side effect
PDDs – pervasive developmental disorders

INTRODUCTION

This chapter provides an overview of the particular issues related to the prescription and use of psychotropic medications in a number of special groups including pregnant and breastfeeding women, children and adolescents, older persons and Indigenous peoples. Psychotropic medications remain the mainstay of treatment for psychiatric disorders but have special considerations when used with these groups of people. In particular, the specific vulnerability of representatives of these groups renders them part of a special group for whom great care must be taken where psychotropic medications are concerned. The chapter begins with the use of these medications by pregnant and breastfeeding women. Age-related issues associated with these medications will then be discussed with a particular focus on children, adolescents and the older person. Finally, issues related to the use of psychotropic medications by Indigenous people will be addressed.

THE PRESCRIPTION AND USE OF PSYCHOTROPIC MEDICATIONS DURING PREGNANCY

Women with pre-existing mental illnesses become pregnant each year, while others develop a mental illness during pregnancy. Many of these women will require psychotropic medications at some stage during their pregnancy. However, the need to balance the risk to the unborn baby and the risk of relapse or deterioration for the woman during pregnancy and in the immediate post-partum period raises significant concerns regarding the prescription and use of psychotropic medications (McCauley-Elsom & Kulkarni 2007). Psychotropic medications, including the newer second generation antipsychotics, are commonly prescribed for women who experience psychoses during pregnancy or the immediate post-partum period (Webb et al 2004). They have not yet been proven safe in pregnancy and their use in pregnancy is not based on evidence from randomised clinical trials (Usher et al 2005). However, perinatal mental health disorders are now a leading cause of maternal morbidity and mortality during pregnancy (Oates 2003), which must be weighed against the risks of prenatal exposure to drugs, including problems such as premature labour, low birth weight, smaller head circumference and inferior functional assessments in the newborn (Viguera & Cohen 1998). Untreated mental disorder has been linked to higher suicide rates, maternal malnutrition and refusal or inability to join in prenatal care activities. Further, these women are often more likely to be without partners or support networks and may hold negative attitudes to pregnancy. Research has shown there is a higher likelihood of developing a psychotic illness following childbirth than at other times during a woman's life and that pre-existing conditions tend to worsen during pregnancy. For example, women with schizophrenia and bipolar disorder are considered to have a 50% risk of recurrence during pregnancy and in the immediate post-partum period (Yaeger et al 2006). Therefore, health professionals caring for pregnant women face the challenge of minimising the risks to the unborn baby while ensuring the safety and wellbeing of the mother. Clinicians and consumers must face the reality that decisions to use or not use psychotropic medications during pregnancy pose threats to both the mother and the baby and that decisions about what constitutes reasonable risk must be a shared decision between the health professional team and the woman. This of course requires that the woman and her partner be informed and included in all decision-making events (see Thinking challenge 7.1).

THINKING CHALLENGE 7.1

McCauley-Elsom and Kulkarni (2007) provide an overview of a case study of a 36-year-old mother of three with a 5-year history of schizophrenia who was pregnant for the fourth time. The woman was well during her pregnancy and continued to take prescribed risperidone and consulted her GP regularly, with whom she had a very good rapport. At 37 weeks, labour was induced due to concerns regarding the baby's failure to grow. She gave birth to a 2.2 kg female who was transferred to a special care nursery due to feeding and thermoregulation problems as well as hyperbilirubinaemia. The baby was discharged to the mother at 6 weeks. At 12 weeks postnatal, the woman attended a new GP for an unstated reason, and the doctor recommended she cease all medications. As a result, the woman's mental state deteriorated and she was admitted to an inpatient mental health unit 5 weeks later and separated from her baby.

QUESTIONS:
» What went wrong here?
» Who could have helped prevent the outcome in this case?
» How can we ensure this type of event does not occur in the future? Remember to consider all health professionals involved and the need for collaboration between health team members.
» Take the time to access and read the entire case study contained in this paper.

Evidence of the teratogenic effects of psychotropic medications is mixed, and their use during pregnancy is a concern because of the exposure of the fetus to an increased risk of congenital malformation. Psychotropic medications readily cross the placenta. The major time of danger for such exposure is the first trimester, although the first 8 weeks appear to be the most significant. Risks from in-utero exposure include spontaneous abortion, structural malformations, carcinogenesis, intrauterine growth retardation, immediate neonatal effects, withdrawal symptoms and behavioural toxicity (Trixler & Tenyi 1997).

USE OF ANTIPSYCHOTICS DURING PREGNANCY
Higher potency first generation antipsychotics such as haloperidol have not been associated with any increased risk of congenital malformations. Low potency first generation antispychotics, such as chlorpromazine, are usually

not prescribed due to concerns about side effects such as hypotension and their association with a slightly higher risk of malformations (Grover et al 2006). Evidence of a perinatal syndrome associated with first generation antipsychotics has been described. These babies demonstrate symptoms of respiratory depression, difficulty feeding, 'floppy baby' syndrome, hypertonicity, sluggish primitive reflexes, extrapyramidal symptoms, tremor, abnormal movements, irritability and agitation. However, the symptoms tend to dissipate within a few days (Yaeger et al 2006). Second generation antipsychotics, rapidly becoming the medication of choice for many people with schizophrenia, do not tend to have some of the side effects of the older, first generation antipsychotics and appear to result in better short- and long-term responses. However, the appropriateness of their use in pregnancy remains unresolved as the limited number of studies is currently inadequate to determine their safety. Therefore, pregnant women prescribed these medications are usually changed to a first generation antipsychotic during pregnancy (Grover et al 2006, Ward & Wisner 2007). A recent study of second generation antipsychotic medications in pregnant women, however, found no statistical differences in the rates of miscarriage, stillbirth, prematurity, congenital malformations and perinatal syndromes in relation to healthy comparison subjects. The study did find an increased rate of babies with low birth weight and, in the mothers, higher body mass index and a greater number of elective abortions. There are concerns that clozapine may be associated with a high rate of congenital malformations. Additional concerns include the known risks of agranulocytosis and orthostatic hypotension associated with clozapine use, which may also have serious effects on the unborn fetus (Yaeger et al 2006).

USE OF MEDICATIONS FOR DEPRESSION AND BIPOLAR DISORDER DURING PREGNANCY

The efficacies of medications used to treat depression and mania have also been studied. There have been concerns about the association between prenatal exposure to lithium and the risk of major congenital abnormalities for more than four decades. Congenital abnormalities recorded include cardiovascular malformations (particularly Ebstein's anomaly), large for gestational age infants, anencephaly and oromandibular-limb hypogenesis. Other risks include muscular hypotonia with impaired breathing and cyanosis (often referred to as 'floppy baby' syndrome), isolated cases of hypothyroidism, nephrogenic diabetes insipidus and polyhydramnios (Grover et al 2006, Ward & Wisner 2007). However, lithium is by far the safest of the anti-manic medications available for use in pregnancy (Ward & Wisner 2007). Compared to lithium, anticonvulsants used to treat mania pose a much more serious threat and should be avoided wherever possible during pregnancy. Carbamazepine has been associated with craniofacial abnormalities, microcephaly, growth retardation, spina bifida, cardiac abnormalities, fingernail hyperplasia and developmental delay. Valproate has been associated with neural tube deficits (particularly those that occur within the first month of gestation), hydrocephalus, cardiovascular malformations, limb defects, genital anomalies and intrauterine growth retardation. The use of valproate near the time of delivery also causes problems for the newborn infant such as jitteriness, feeding difficulties, irritability, heart rate deceleration, hypoglycaemia and abnormal tone (Grover et al 2006, Ward & Wisner 2007). Prenatal use of tricyclic antidepressants or the newer selective serotonin reuptake inhibitors (SSRIs) used to treat depression does not appear to increase the risk of congenital abnormalities although these agents can cause minor complications if used close to the time of delivery. For example, studies have found evidence of poor neonatal adaptation syndrome, which includes tremors, jitteriness, shivering, feeding or digestive problems and respiratory distress. These problems were, however, relatively minor and short-lived (Way 2007). In general, the SSRIs are preferred to the tricyclic antidepressants (Sved Williams 2007). The only antidepressant that may be unsuitable for use during pregnancy is paroxetine. Recent research indicates that there may be a small risk of congenital abnormalities, especially cardiac defects, related to the use of paroxetine during pregnancy (Way 2007). To date the evidence for venlafaxine indicates it is safe to use during pregnancy but, although it is not associated with a higher rate of birth defects, it has been linked to increased rates of spontaneous abortion. According to the data available on the use of mirtazapine during pregnancy, it should be avoided (Sved Williams 2007). Monoamine oxidase inhibitors (MAOIs) are considered best avoided because of the risk of hypertensive crises.

USE OF OTHER PSYCHOTROPICS DURING PREGNANCY

The benzodiazepines, psychotropic medications commonly used as an adjunct treatment for mood stabilisation, anxiety, agitation and sleep disorders, also readily cross the placenta and may pose a risk to the fetus. The risk of malformations from this class of medication is highest during the first 8 weeks of pregnancy. Medications of this type administered close to the time of delivery have also been linked to fetal dependence and withdrawal symptoms. The use of diazepam during pregnancy is considered safe, and evidence indicates that the use of this medication during pregnancy causes no harm to the fetus (Iqbal et al 2002). The use of other benzodiazepine medications such as clonazepam, lorazepam and alprazolam has, however, been linked to serious congenital abnormalities and thus should be avoided during the first trimester of pregnancy (Grover et al 2006).

Usher, Foster and MacNamara (2005) proposed guidelines for the use of antipsychotic medication by women who are pregnant (see Box 7.1) or breastfeeding. These include the following:

- Antipsychotics, including depot injections, should be avoided in the first trimester.
- Women using second generation antipsychotics should change to first generation antipsychotics as soon as pregnancy is diagnosed.
- Pregnant and breastfeeding women should be prescribed the lowest possible dose.
- Depot injections should be avoided with breastfeeding women.
- Only infants born at full term should be exposed to the potential to ingest medication via breast milk (see Thinking challenge 7.2).

BOX 7.1 – GUIDELINES FOR MANAGING PREGNANT WOMEN TAKING ANTIPSYCHOTIC MEDICATIONS

» Conduct regular comprehensive assessments of the women
» Avoid antipsychotics in the first trimester if possible
» Where possible, change prescriptions from atypical antipsychotics to typical antipsychotics during the first trimester
» Always prescribe and administer the lowest possible dose of psychotropic medications
» Avoid depot injections during pregnancy
» Provide evidence-based educational information to the woman and her partner
» Engage the woman and her partner in decision making
» Document and report all relevant findings

(Adapted from Usher et al 2005, p 717)

THINKING CHALLENGE 7.2

Many community-based health professionals may be involved in advising a pregnant woman about the issues of taking psychotropic medications during pregnancy. How do you think you would advise someone in this situation? What are the main issues to be considered when weighing up the risks to the mother and fetus and how would you relate these in your clinical interview? List the special issues that may be relevant to your clinical role versus other members of the health care team.

Given the risks associated with the use of psychotropic medications during pregnancy, it is imperative that members of the health care team are aware of the medications that must be avoided and work together to ensure all other available strategies have been explored before psychotropic medications are prescribed (see Clinical alert 7.1). If prescribed, the lowest dose possible for the shortest period of time is recommended, and regular, individual assessments of the risks and benefits that fully involve the woman and her family should be made. Monitoring of the woman at regular intervals during the pregnancy and after the birth is important to ensure the ongoing wellbeing of both the mother and baby.

CLINICAL ALERT 7.1 – MEDICATIONS THAT SHOULD BE AVOIDED DURING PREGNANCY
Antipsychotics Clozapine
Antidepressants Paroxetine Mirtazapine All monoamine oxidase inhibitors (MAOIs)
Antimanics All anticonvulsants used for mood stabilisation
Benzodiazepines Clonazepam, lorazepam, alprazolam

THE USE OF PSYCHOTROPIC MEDICATIONS WHEN BREASTFEEDING

Women with pre-existing mental disorders may continue to require the prescription and administration of psychotropic medications after childbirth. Evidence indicates that 10–15% of all postpartum women will develop some form of mental disorder (Winans 2001, Oates 2003), and those women with a pre-existing condition are at a higher risk of developing a relapse in the postnatal period (Ilett et al 2004). These women may also require psychotropic medications. Of relevance here is the relation to the woman's decision to breastfeed her infant, a normal and highly recommended practice (Malone et al 2004) whose benefits are well documented. The relationship between breastfeeding and mental disorders, especially postnatal depression, is complex. Women who develop depression are considered more likely to cease breastfeeding. However the converse is also true as women who establish and maintain breastfeeding are found to be less likely to become depressed than women who experience difficulties with breastfeeding (Sved Williams 2007). Decisions to prescribe or administer psychotropic medications should weigh up the woman's preference to breastfeed and the risk to the infant versus the benefit to the mother. The decisions should be made in a collaborative way, including all members of the health care team, after the woman and her partner/family have been fully informed of the risks and benefits of the medication.

Overall, the available research on the safety of psychotropic medications when breastfeeding is limited and fraught with confounding variables. Most psychotropic medications pass into breast milk but there is a significant variation in the amount actually received by the infant. The plasma level of the medication in the neonate involves various factors such as the medication level at birth (when the mother was taking the medication prior to delivery), the relative degree of transfer of the medication to the breast milk, the half-life of the drug, the protein binding ability of the drug, time of peak serum concentration in the mother and its relation to feeding and the amount of milk produced and ingested by the infant (Hale 2004, Usher & Foster 2006). We do know that the transfer of psychotropic medications to breast milk is less efficient than placental transfer (i.e., blood-to-blood in pregnancy versus blood-to-milk-to-gut-to-blood in breastfeeding) (Stowe 2007). Therefore, the risk of these medications to the breastfed newborn may be lower than during pregnancy but a risk nevertheless.

USE OF ANTIPSYCHOTICS DURING BREASTFEEDING

Available evidence indicates that all antipsychotic medications are excreted into breast milk (see Clinical alert 7.2). Lactation studies with first generation antipsychotic medications have consistently reported low milk to plasma transfer levels (< 1) (Jain & Lacy 2005). However, it has been recommended that the phenothiazine group of first generation antipsychotics be avoided wherever possible because of their potential for neonatal apnoea and sedation (Hale 2004). Clozapine, found at high levels in infants at the time of delivery but significantly reduced after 1 week, is not recommended during breastfeeding. Case reports have identified problems such as sedation, cardiovascular instability and agranulocytosis (Jain & Lacy 2005). Studies of the effects of olanzapine on 21 breast-fed infants revealed five reports of adverse effects including jaundice, cardiomegaly, heart murmur, shaking, lethargy, poor sucking, protruding tongue, rashes, diarrhoea and sleeping problems. Studies of risperidone and quetiapine have shown no adverse effects so far (Ernst & Goldberg 2002).

CLINICAL ALERT 7.2 – USE OF ANTIPSYCHOTICS WHEN BREASTFEEDING

All antipsychotic medications are excreted into breast milk and therefore have some impact on the breastfed neonate.

This is important to remember when advising the mother and her partner.

USE OF ANTIDEPRESSANTS DURING BREASTFEEDING

Overall, there have been relatively few studies demonstrating adverse effects in infants exposed to antidepressants via breast milk. The tricyclic antidepressants, now only used minimally, are relatively safe to use when breastfeeding. The SSRIs are commonly the first choice for pregnant and breastfeeding women because they tend to cause fewer autonomic and other side effects and because the rate of transfer to, and uptake by, the baby is relatively low (Hale 2004). Venlafaxine is, however, thought to accumulate in the breastfed baby so it is therefore not recommended for prolonged use (Sved Williams 2007). Case reports of adverse effects from trazodone and bupropion have also been reported but it is considered too soon to draw any firm conclusions about the safety of those medications during breastfeeding. It has been recommended that fluoxetine (due to its long half-life) and high doses of citalopram (because of high plasma and breast milk concentrations) be avoided except in women who have demonstrated good outcomes with the medication during pregnancy. The research to date shows low or undetectable levels with sertraline, paroxetine and fluvoxamine (Payne 2007). It is important to weigh up the benefits of the antidepressant medications against the risks of untreated postnatal depression. As well as the risk to the mother, failure to adequately treat maternal depression can result in poor mother–baby bonding, potential effects on the child's intelligence level and delayed development (Payne 2007) (see Chat box 7.1).

CHAT BOX 7.1

Exposure of a child to postpartum depression should be considered an exposure in the same way that taking an antidepressant while breastfeeding is an exposure.

(Payne 2007, p 1330)

This is an interesting quote. What is the point being made and why has the author felt the need to make it? Consider how it relates to decisions women and their partners must make in these situations. What are the particular implications for your clinical role?

USE OF OTHER PSYCHOTROPICS DURING BREASTFEEDING

Lithium may have been unfairly rated as unsuitable for use when breastfeeding infants due to the potential for adverse effects (Stowe 2007). Recent studies found serum lithium levels in nursing infants to be low and well tolerated. Further, there were no significant adverse clinical or behavioural effects noted (Viguera et al 2007). Lithium is thus considered relatively safe in compliant mothers, but the infants must receive regular monitoring for serum lithium concentrations as well as renal and thyroid function (Sved Williams 2007). The anticonvulsants used to treat mood disorders, carbamazepine and valproate, are also considered safe for use in breastfeeding women.

The use of benzodiazepines while breastfeeding is not recommended (see Box 7.2). These medications have been found to accumulate in breast milk and in the infant. While single doses of the medication may be acceptable, ongoing use should be avoided (Usher & Foster 2006). Signs of toxicity include lethargy, hypotonia, poor feeding and sedation.

BOX 7.2 – GUIDELINES FOR MANAGING BREASTFEEDING WOMEN AND NEONATES WHEN ANTIPSYCHOTIC MEDICATIONS ARE PRESCRIBED

» Do a comprehensive assessment of mother and neonate at birth and/or at commencement of breastfeeding at regular intervals
» Provide mother and partner with evidence-based educational materials
» Encourage collaborative decision making where possible
» Monitor neonates closely while the mother is taking psychotropic medications
» At the first sign of toxicity in the neonate, terminate breastfeeding and refer
» Warn mothers against polypharmacy, especially taking additional over-the-counter medications while breastfeeding

---

(Adapted from Usher et al 2005, p 717)

THE USE OF PSYCHOTROPIC MEDICATIONS IN CHILDREN AND ADOLESCENTS

During the past few years we have witnessed a substantial rise in the use of psychotropic medications in children and adolescents without a corresponding rise in the incidence of psychiatric disorders. The brain continues to develop as the child grows, possibly accounting for the different presentation of symptoms of mental illness in children and adolescents compared to adults. For example, the underlying biological substrate for depression might change while the psychological substrate remains the same. It cannot be assumed, therefore, that because a medication works with adults, it will work in the same way for children. Further, it is important to recognise that children and adolescents should not be viewed as 'little adults' but rather treated as distinct groups, each with their own unique characteristics and, thus, response to drug therapy (Lakhan & Hagger-Johnson 2007). As children and adolescents experience psychiatric disorders differently to adults, this must be considered when planning appropriate treatments (Bolfek et al 2006).

The issue of safety with regard to the use of psychotropic medications is very important with children. The developing brain, which is anatomically vulnerable, is programmed to mature in a particular sequence. To date, the long-term effects of psychotropic medications on the developing brain have not been determined (Lakhan & Hagger-Johnson 2007). Therefore the use of psychotropic medications with this group is extremely complex and must be undertaken judiciously. Ideally, non-pharmacological strategies should be employed prior to resorting to the use of psychotropic medications. In a recent New Zealand study of children receiving psychotropic medication, most children surveyed were treated with risperidone, but the findings suggested some psychotropic medications were prescribed for disorders outside what is currently recommended (see Chat box 7.2). For example, second generation antipsychotics were prescribed for sleep disorder in children (Harrison-Woolrych et al 2007), indicating that the use of the medications may not have kept pace with the available evidence, especially related to safety (Jensen et al 2007).

CHAT BOX 7.2

... the use of these agents has often surpassed the available evidence ...

(Jensen et al 2007, p 105)

This is a serious concern given the impact of the medications on the developing brain and the limited data on adverse effects, especially in the longer term.

USE OF ANTIPSYCHOTICS IN CHILDREN AND ADOLESCENTS

Second generation antipsychotics are now used to treat a range of mental health disorders that occur in childhood and adolescence. Pharmacological treatment tends to be a last resort for disruptive behavioural disorders (DBDs) (e.g., conduct disorder, such as destructiveness and violence, and oppositional defiant disorder, such as rule breaking), pervasive developmental disorders (PDDs) (e.g., autism, Asperger's syndrome) and tic disorders (e.g., Tourette's syndrome, chronic motor and vocal tic disorder, transient tic disorder) (see Thinking challenge 7.3). Non-pharmacological interventions such as psychosocial therapy or family therapy tend to be the preferred first line of treatment for these disorders. However, if the symptoms are severe and fail to respond to non-pharmacological treatment, or interfere with family, social or academic functioning, second generation antipsychotic medications will be prescribed and trialled. The second generation antipsychotics, such as risperidone and olanzapine, will usually be prescribed because of their more tolerable adverse effect profile when compared to the first generation antispsychotics (see Clinical alert 7.3).

Schizophrenia and bipolar disorder are more often diagnosed in adolescents or young adults rather than children. In children the rate of occurrence of schizophrenia has been reported as 0.01%. Second generation antipsychotics have been reported to have a higher efficacy than the first

THINKING CHALLENGE 7.3

Some have said that children have no reason to develop depression or anxiety. Do you believe this is true, or do you think children experience similar stressors to adults? If you answered yes, list the stressors particular to children and adolescents.

CLINICAL ALERT 7.3 – MEDICATIONS FOR AGITATION/AGGRESSION IN CHILDREN/ADOLESCENTS

At times, children and adolescents will display agitation and/or aggression that will require intervention. Pharmacological interventions in this case must be tailored to the special needs of the child, taking account of their age. The administration of a benzodiazepine may be the safer choice but can lead to 'rebound irritability'. Diazepam is the preferred oral benzodiazepine and dosage must be adjusted for weight and individual response. Smaller doses of PRN (as needed) antipsychotics may be used in preference to, or in combination with, the benzodiazepine. Suitable oral antipsychotics include haloperidol (1–2 mg), dispersible and liquid preparations of risperidone (1–2 mg) and olanzapine (2.5–10 mg). Intramuscular options include haloperidol (1–2 mg) and olanzapine (1–2 mg).

(Adapted from Tiffin 2007, p 180)

generation antipsychotics when used to treat psychoses in children and adolescents, and risperidone, olanzapine and clozapine are commonly prescribed (Jensen et al 2007, Tiffin 2007). The older first generation antipsychotics are now used only to treat children and adolescents when the response to second generation antipsychotic medications is poor, or for use as a treatment for agitation or distress or when a depot preparation is required (Tiffin 2007) (see Thinking challenge 7.4).

THINKING CHALLENGE 7.4

Non-pharmacological treatments play an important role in the management of psychiatric disorders in children and adolescents – considered by many health professionals as a more important role than medications. Read the article by Tiffin (2007) and outline the types of therapies used and your views on the major benefits of using alternative treatments to medications.

Adverse effects in paediatric patients treated with risperidone, clozapine or olanzapine, in both short- and long-term studies, include somnolence and weight gain. Extrapyramidal side effects (EPSEs), in particular abnormal involuntary movements, have been detected in children and adolescents in the first few days of treatment with antipsychotics, as well as during short- and long-term treatments. The abnormal movements include jerky movements of the fingers and wrist, jerky protrusions and mild writhing movements of the tongue, blinking and other tic-like movements of the neck and arms (Laita et al 2007). Serious haematological effects have been reported with clozapine, and there is evidence that treatment with ziprasidone can lead to serious electrocardiographical changes associated with increased risk of arrhythmia and sudden death. Longer term studies have so far failed to find evidence, at least with risperidone, that second generation antispychotics have a negative impact on cognitive functioning, growth or sexual maturation (Jensen et al 2007).

Weight gain is viewed as a class effect although it is most pronounced during the initial phases of treatment and is more evident with clozapine and olanzapine (see Thinking challenge 7.5). One recent study reported weight gain in 11% of the participating children, although reports of weight gain as high as 36% have been associated with the use of risperidone, as reported elsewhere (Harrison-Woolrych et al 2007). Metabolic and endocrine side effects, increases in serum cholesterol and LDL levels and weight gain are common in adults, which makes the use of these medications in children and adolescents even more of a concern. Limited data are currently available to help unravel the links between obesity and the associated cluster of metabolic events, such as metabolic syndrome and diabetes (Jensen et al 2007).

THINKING CHALLENGE 7.5

Consider the impact weight gain may have on a child or adolescent who already feels embarrassed because of their psychiatric disorder and try to imagine how that might further impact on their social and emotional development and relationships. List some of the main issues you believe should be considered when using these medications with this group.

USE OF MEDICATIONS FOR DEPRESSION AND BIPOLAR DISORDER IN CHILDREN AND ADOLESCENTS

Mood disorders in children and adolescents are common and bipolar disorder, once considered rare in children, is now quite commonly diagnosed. Depression is a common disorder in children (2–5%) and increases dramatically in incidence as children enter adolescence (Bolfek et al 2006), perhaps explained by the increasing stressors faced by adolescents. Children and adolescents with depression present differently from adults. They are more likely to present with irritability and other negative emotions such as anxiety and anger. Depression in adolescents rarely manifests as a solitary problem but rather occurs as part of a complex pattern of behaviour that makes diagnosis much more difficult (Bolfek et al 2006). Antidepressants should only be prescribed with extreme caution in this group due to the risk of precipitating affective disturbance (Tiffin 2007) (see Box 7.3). If antidepressants are prescribed, SSRIs should be used in preference to the tricyclic antidepressants which, although shown to be effective in adults, have failed to demonstrate efficacy in children and are associated with potentially life-threatening adverse events (see Clinical alert 7.4). The SSRI fluoxetine is considered the first choice for depression in adolescence and is also used for children with obsessive–compulsive disorder (note the Drug interaction box below). The SSRIs are generally well tolerated in children and side effects, if experienced, tend to be minimal and usually subside within 1–2 weeks (see Table 7.1 for dosing ranges). Adverse effects most often experienced include headache, abdominal pain, nausea, diarrhoea, sleep changes and jitteriness or agitation, but can also include diaphoresis, akathisia, bruising and changes in sexual function (Bolfek et al 2006). More serious side effects have however been associated with SSRIs in children. Serotonin syndrome and extrapyramidal symptoms as well as tics and myoclonus have been described in children, adolescents and adults. An amotivational syndrome, linked to the use of SSRIs in adults, has also been observed in children and adolescents and is thought to be the result of dopamine inhibition (Hammerness et al 2006). If antidepressant therapy is prescribed, the child or adolescent must be closely observed for signs of worsening or suicidality, which is still considered a risk with this treatment (Bolfek et al 2006), and for other signs of adverse effects.

BOX 7.3 – MANAGEMENT OF CHILDREN AND ADOLESCENTS TAKING ANTIDEPRESSANTS

» Adjust the dose for variables such as age, body weight, pubertal status and family history of drug response
» Observe closely for signs of clinical worsening, suicidality or unusual behaviours
» Educate families and caregivers regarding the need for close monitoring
» Educate regarding expected side effects and their management
» Ensure weekly face-to-face contact with the health care team during the first 4 weeks of treatment
» Arrange visits every other week for the next 4 weeks, then taper off to every 12 weeks
» Continue treatment for 6 to 9 months and then maintenance for up to 5 years
» Time the gradual tapering of the medication, taking psychosocial stressors into account

(Hammerness et al 2006, p 160)

CLINICAL ALERT 7.4 – SSRIs AND MOOD STABILISATION

Switching implies a switch from one mood state to another, such as from depression to mania, while taking an antidepressant such as an SSRI. It has been found to occur in up to 5% of a study sample, and children aged 10 to 14 are considered to be at highest risk. If this occurs it precludes the use of SSRIs until adequate mood stabilisation can be achieved.

(Hammerness et al 2006, p 162)

DRUG INTERACTION – MAOIs, SSRIs

Monamine oxidase inhibitors (MAOIs) must not be given within 5 weeks of discontinuation of fluoxetine or within 2 weeks of discontinuation of other SSRIs to avoid serotonin syndrome. The converse is also true.

TABLE 7.1 – DOSING RANGE FOR SSRIs IN PAEDIATRIC PRACTICE

	Starting dose, mg		
Drug	Pre-adolescent	Adolescent	Typical dose range, mg
Fluoxetine*	2.5–10	10–20	10–80
Sertraline	12.5–25	25–50	50–200
Fluvoxamine	12.5–25	25–50	50–300
Paroxetine**	2.5–10	10	10–60
Citalopram	2.5–10	10–20	10–60

*Oral concentrate is available.
**Oral suspension is available.

(Adapted from Hammerness et al 2005, p 161)

The precise evidence of bipolar spectrum in children and adolescents is unclear and, even though childhood onset was once considered rare, some studies suggest it may be as high in adolescents as in adults. When symptoms present before the age of 12, they may be confused with ADHD. The clinical presentation of this familial condition is different in children and young adolescents but often similar in late adolescence. In the pre-pubertal child, there may be clear but brief adult-like episodes shifting in rapid cycles of several hours to days. Children are most likely to present with irritability, mood lability, affective 'storms', continuous mixed depressive and manic symptoms, aggressive or explosive behaviour or impulsive and distractible behaviour without clearly delineated episodes (Bolfek et al 2006). Children with these disorders experience difficulty with academic success and interpersonal relationships and are at much greater risk for substance misuse, legal difficulties, increased suicidal behaviour and hospitalisation (Hamrin & Pachler 2007). Treatment of these episodes is complex and often lifelong. Medications that have been found useful in adults have been used with modified strategies in the younger age groups. Even though lithium has been used successfully for the treatment of mania in younger people, it is rarely employed with children and adolescents because of the risk of toxicity (Tiffin 2007). If used, the target dose is 30 mg/kg/day in 3 to 4 divided doses with serum levels of 0.9–1.1 mEq/L recommended (Bolfek et al 2006). The anticonvulsants have also been used in the treatment of mania in children and adolescents. Valproate, commonly used in children for whom lithium is not recommended, has demonstrated response rates of 46–80% and is well tolerated when combined with other medications (Hamrin & Pachler 2007). Side effects include nausea, sedation, weight gain and development of polycystic ovary syndrome (Bolfek et al 2006). Antipsychotics, especially the second generation, may also be prescribed for the treatment of mania but, if used in combination, the dose must be reduced. Quetiapine, risperidone and olanzapine have been effective in the short-term management of bipolar disorder in children (Hamrin & Pachler 2007) (see Box 7.4).

BOX 7.4 – MANAGEMENT OF ANTIPSYCHOTIC SIDE EFFECTS IN CHILDREN AND ADOLESCENTS

» Use the lowest effective dose
» Change medications if required
» Manage akathisia via short-term use of benzodiazepines
» Provide nutritional advice and exercise education to reduce the likelihood of weight gain
» Manage hypersalivation caused by clozapine with antimuscarinic agents such as oxybutynin

---

(Tiffin 2007)

USE OF MEDICATIONS FOR ATTENTION DEFICIT DISORDERS IN CHILDREN AND ADOLESCENTS

Attention deficit disorder (ADD) and attention deficit/hyperactivity disorder (ADHD) are also disorders of childhood. These disorders cause significant alterations in emotional, behavioural and cognitive functioning and can have significant economic, educational, social and health costs for the affected person and their families. The prevalence worldwide is estimated at 5–10% of children and 4% of adults (Faraone et al 2003, Faraone 2004). While the conditions generally develop during childhood and adolescence, they may persist into adulthood.

The clinical manifestations of these conditions are summarised in Table 7.2. An important feature of these conditions is co-morbidity. People with attention deficits can also show mood, anxiety, conduct and tic disorders as well as substance misuse disorders. Genetic factors are strongly implicated in the development of these attention disorders. Studies of twins have demonstrated a mean heritability of 77% for ADHD (Faraone et al 2005, Spencer et al 2007). Other factors that have been suggested include diet and the levels of food additives, exposure to lead in the environment, smoking and alcohol use during pregnancy, low birth weight, complications of pregnancy and delivery and an aggregate of psychosocial adversity factors (Spencer et al 2007).

TABLE 7.2 – THE COMMON CLINICAL MANIFESTATIONS OF ADD/ADHD	
Symptoms of attentional deficit	Symptoms of hyperactivity
Inattentiveness Poor concentration Easily distracted Impulsiveness Difficulty in focusing on one task for a prolonged period	Restlessness Fidgety behaviour Excessive talkativeness Irritability Moodiness Aimlessness Poor self-esteem Difficulty in adjusting socially

The pathophysiology of attention deficit disorders remains unclear. Structurally, changes within the prefrontal cortex have been proposed. The dorsolateral prefrontal cortex (DLPFC), orbitofrontal region and the anterior cingulate cortex have been implicated. The DLPFC is involved in organised thought, planning, working memory and attention. The orbitofrontal region plays a role in social disinhibition and impulse control. The anterior cingulate is involved in attention. The corpus striatum, corpus callosum and cerebellum have also been implicated in the pathophysiology of these conditions. Neuroimaging studies have revealed smaller volumes in these regions and in total brain volumes in people affected by ADHD. Alterations in the communication between these regions and the cortex, or between hemispheres, may account for the symptoms of ADHD and ADD.

Chemical imbalances in dopaminergic and noradrenergic brain systems are considered to account for the symptomology of these attention disorders. A change in the chemical modulation of pathways between the prefrontal cortex and subcortical structures is thought to underlie the problem. A relative deficiency in these catecholamine transmitters may lead to less than normal waking inhibition by the prefrontal cortex on subcortical and other brain structures, resulting in inattention and hyperactivity (Cabral 2006).

The decision to use medications as the treatment for ADD and ADHD in children is not easy for health professionals and parents. However, if pharmacological treatment is chosen as the best option, a range of medications can be used. The mainstay of treatment for ADD and ADHD has been the central nervous system stimulants, methylphenidate and dexamphetamine. These drugs can rapidly enhance attention, reduce hyperactivity and improve social behaviour and cognition. At first glance it appears counter-intuitive to use stimulants to control hyperactivity. However, these drugs do offer some relief for the majority of sufferers. The CNS stimulants are thought to increase synaptic amine transmitter activity, especially that of dopamine and noradrenaline and, to a lesser extent, serotonin. These actions enhance amine neurotransmission. Both of these drugs bind to and block the presynaptic dopamine transporter protein (see Fig 7.1). Methylphenidate exerts this action predominately in the prefrontal cortex and corpus striatum, key areas implicated in the pathophysiology of these conditions. Methylphenidate has a similar action on the presynaptic noradrenaline transporter protein in the CNS. Dexamphetamine inhibits presynaptic noradrenaline reuptake and enhances the release of dopamine presynaptically.

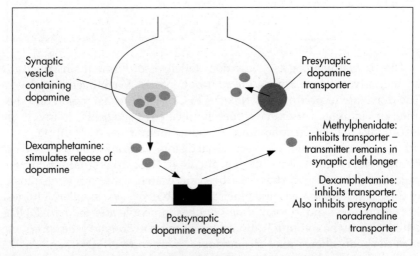

Figure 7.1 – Mechanisms of action of the CNS stimulants at the synapse
An action potential triggers the release of the transmitter into the synaptic cleft, where it interacts with the receptor producing activation of the CNS pathway. Presynaptic transmitter transporter inactivates the transmitter action by returning the chemical messenger back to the presynaptic terminal. CNS stimulants increase synaptic transmitter levels, enhancing the action of the chemical messenger on the pathway.

As stimulants, these drugs possess significant potential for addiction to develop so their use needs to be closely monitored. Common adverse effects associated with CNS stimulation include insomnia, restlessness, appetite suppression and gastrointestinal disturbances. Cardiovascular reactions need to be monitored and include cardiac dysrhythmias, palpitations and alterations in blood pressure. A novel non-stimulant agent, atomoxetine, has recently been introduced into the region for use in the management of ADHD. It inhibits the presynaptic noradrenaline transporter protein in the prefrontal cortex. It also affects serotonin and, to a lesser extent, dopamine reuptake in the CNS. Interestingly, it can stimulate 5-HT$_2$ and GABA$_A$ receptors within the CNS and these effects may also contribute to the therapeutic action of this agent. Common adverse effects include hypertension, tachycardia, appetite suppression, sedation, nausea, vomiting and abdominal pain.

Greydanus et al (2007) have reviewed other drugs that are considered useful in ADD and ADHD. These include antidepressants, alpha-2 agonists and noradrenaline reuptake inhibitors. As the tricyclic antidepressants block noradrenaline and serotonin reuptake, they are considered to be of some use in ADHD. However, they are not as efficacious as the CNS stimulants and their use may be limited by the severity of their adverse effect profile (see Ch 2). Bupropion, whose primary indication is in the management of nicotine addiction (see Ch 6), was first developed as an antidepressant. It can be used in ADD and ADHD to reduce irritability and improve attention. Its mechanism of action is to inhibit the reuptake of noradrenaline and dopamine and this is consistent with the hypothesis that enhanced catecholamine neurotransmission is of therapeutic benefit in these disorders. The sedative action of the alpha-2 agonist clonidine is considered useful in counteracting insomnia in children with ADHD.

Drugs represent only one part of the management of these conditions. Psychotherapy and access to support groups and training programs for parents, teachers and consumers alike can assist in the identification and management of early disruptive behaviours before they escalate.

ETHICAL ISSUES ASSOCIATED WITH THE PRESCRIPTION AND USE OF PSYCHOTROPIC MEDICATIONS IN CHILDREN AND ADOLESCENTS

Many health professionals, ethicists and others have expressed the view that psychotropic medications should not be prescribed for use in children (Lacramioara & Arnold 2007, Healy 2005) (see Chat box 7.3). Children and adolescents with a psychiatric disorder are considered a vulnerable group by virtue of both psychiatric diagnosis and developmental stage (Solyom & Moreno 2005), thus a careful approach must be taken to their treatment. Ethicists and others have therefore raised concerns over issues related to the use of psychotropic medications in this group, particularly because of the greater risk of drug toxicity, the side effect profiles of the drugs (especially the increased risk of suicidality, weight gain and EPSEs) and the lack of valid evidence to support their efficacy and safety in children. The results of long-lasting side effects such as polycystic ovary and the impact on the developing child versus the need to relieve the distress of the mental disorder have also been debated. The growing trend of prescribing psychotropic medications for children with a range of disorders is alarming and is now recognised as a significant concern. This is especially relevant to the burgeoning rate of diagnosis of disorders such as ADHD and the associated use of stimulants in children and adolescents.

CHAT BOX 7.3

Unless a child's problem is very severe and/or the child's response to treatment shows very clear and substantial benefits, it would be difficult to justify the use of these drugs in children, other than on a short-term basis.

(Healy 2005, p 125)

This statement sums up the views of many on this topic. Some go further, however, and say that the medications should not be used under any circumstances.

To date, there is little evidence to support long-term safe use of these medications in the developing brain, and only limited studies have been conducted to determine appropriate dosages and to predict the side effect profile and response in younger children. There are also concerns that the efficacy and safety of these medications have in the past been overstated and, even worse, there is evidence that some drug companies have deliberately left out information on the hazards of the treatment or suppressed raw data that may have made a difference to a study outcome (Healy 2005, Perlis et al 2005). Others claim that children are 'therapeutic orphans' because information related to the efficacy and usage of these medications in children has been extrapolated from studies of adults (Lacramioara & Arnold 2007) and, thus, these people argue for the need to conduct research into the effect of psychotropic medications on children and adolescents (see Thinking challenge 7.6).

THINKING CHALLENGE 7.6

» What are the ethical principles that relate to the prescription and use of psychotropic medications with children and adolescents?
» Do the same principles apply to research on the use of these medications with children and adolescents and why/why not?

Concerns with regard to the risks of unethical research or exposure to suboptimal treatment have caused many, including clinicians, ethicists and others, to speak out and raise concerns about the use of psychotropic medications in this group. This is an area that requires further attention in the future, and decisions to conduct further research including children and adolescents must take account of the expressed views and concerns and balance the evidence against what appears to be the best option for the child.

THE USE OF PSYCHOTROPIC MEDICATIONS IN OLDER PERSONS

Older persons represent a rapidly increasing proportion of patients seen in clinical practice and within inpatient facilities. Even though older persons are relatively fit and healthy, many have multiple pathologies that can confound diagnosis. In general, they are known to take more medications than younger people and frequently take more than one medication. Further, older persons experience high rates of mental health disorders including mood and anxiety disorders, bipolar affective disorder, psychotic disorders, depression and dementia. Psychotropic medications have an important role in the management of these disorders and studies indicate that the rates of use of psychotropic medications are high in the older age groups. One person in six aged over 50 years (for women) and over 60 years (for men) has been found to use psychotropic medications of some sort (Empereur et al 2003). The rates of use of psychotropic medications are also high among those in aged care facilities (Malone et al 2007). Previous studies have revealed that more than 40% of persons with dementia living in aged care facilities are prescribed antipsychotics (Alanen et al 2006) (see Thinking challenge 7.7). Men and women over 50 take psychotropic medications to deal with work and health related issues and sleep disorders. The higher use of psychotropics in these age groups has also been linked to widowed and divorced persons over 50 versus married or single and to combinations with alcohol and/or cigarettes (Empereur et al 2003). A recent Australian study (Windle et al 2007) reported that, in a sample of 3970 general practice patients over 65, 625 had at least one benzodiazepine prescription, giving a prevalence of 15.7%, which is similar to the findings of other studies. The research also identified that females were almost twice as likely as males to be prescribed a benzodiazepine and that 45% of the cohort had between two and six prescribing events and 15% had seven or more (Windle et al 2007). These trends raise serious concerns.

Particular care must be taken when psychotropic medications are

---

THINKING CHALLENGE 7.7

Write down some of the factors that might be related to the greater use of psychotropic medications in elderly persons residing in aged care facilities. How does this impact on your current or future role in the health care team?

---

considered for use in this group, however, as older persons are much more vulnerable when it comes to adverse effects and usually require a much lower dose than younger people. Adverse effects are usually much more pronounced in the older person in general because of a decline in physiological response. These problems may stem from inhibition of an already compromised system or organ, or be related to an increased organ sensitivity (Sadavoy 2007). With psychotropic medications, where sedation, orthostatic hypotension and EPSEs are known to be more prominent, management problems can arise (Malone et al 2007). For example, benzodiazepines are more likely to cause dizziness in the older person, which can lead to falls, serious injury (Shupikai Rinomhota & Marshall 2000) and accidents without significantly improving the condition for which they were originally prescribed (Windle et al 2007).

USE OF ANTIDEPRESSANTS IN OLDER PERSONS

Older persons have similar response rates to antidepressants as younger age groups (Hopwood 2007). The more favourable adverse profile of the newer antidepressants, such as the SSRIs and SNRIs, means that they should be the treatment of choice over tricyclics (Hopwood 2007, Sadavoy 2007). However, they do have significant side effects in the older person and must be used with caution. The consumer must be assessed for anxiety and akathisia reactions to the medication and should have sodium levels monitored. Fluoxetine is not recommended for use with older persons because of its long half-life (Sadavoy 2007). Disappointingly, there have been few studies of the efficacy and tolerability of mood stabilisers in older people. Case reports and clinical evidence suggest they are equally effective. Lithium poses a particular problem due to its narrow therapeutic index making it more complex to manage in this age group. It can be used but the older person must be closely monitored for adverse effects. In addition, the consumer and their partner and family should be educated about the common drug interactions, especially with diuretics and non-steroidal anti-inflammatory drugs, ACE inhibitors and metronidazole (Hopwood 2007).

USE OF ANTIPSYCHOTICS IN OLDER PERSONS

First and second generation antipsychotic medications are used to treat various disorders in the older person including psychosis, bipolar affective disorder, delirium and dementia. Increasingly, the second generation or atypical antipsychotics have become more popular because of their reduced rate of EPSEs. However, adverse effects such as antimuscarinic anticholinergic and cardiovascular effects, sedation, tardive dyskinesia, stroke, cardiopulmonary events and death indicate they must be used with extreme caution with the elderly. The effect of sedation in this age group can be extended, increasing the likelihood of falls or other accidents (Malone et al 2007). When used, they should be administered at lower doses than in younger people and titrated over longer periods of time to reach the required dose. In other words, 'start low and go slow' (Malone et al 2007) with older people when prescribing antipsychotics (see Clinical alert 7.5). Persons with dementia have been found to be particularly at risk from these medications and their use is not recommended (Kales et al 2007), an alarming fact given that the rate of prescription is reportedly high for persons with dementia living in aged care facilities (Alanen et al 2006).

Few studies have been conducted on the safety of depot antipsychotics

---

CLINICAL ALERT 7.5 – NEUROLEPTIC MALIGNANT SYNDROME IN THE OLDER PERSON

Even though it is more likely to occur in a younger age group, neuroleptic malignant syndrome (NMS) (outlined in detail in Ch 4) can also affect the older person. The risk is especially high for people with Parkinson's disease or Lewy body dementia. Abrupt withdrawal of antipsychotic medications in this group may induce NMS. Antipsychotic medications should be avoided in these persons if at all possible. If antipsychotic medications must be used, quetiapine and clozapine are the more desirable choices because of their dopamine receptor occupancies.

(Malone et al 2004)

---

for the elderly. Of the traditional or first generation antipsychotic medications, low doses of haloperidol and fluphenazine are the preferred depot antipsychotic for use with the elderly as they tend to cause less sedation, postural hypotension and antimuscarinic anticholinergic effect. Of the second generation antipsychotics, risperidone is the first to be approved as a long-acting injectable. To date it appears to have a favourable safety profile with the older person.

USE OF MEDICATIONS FOR ALZHEIMER'S DISEASE AND DEMENTIA

Cognitive enhancers, used to reduce symptoms and disease progression in Alzheimer's disease (AD), have limited effectiveness yet are seen as the new 'hope' for a better future. Initially the aim was to develop drugs to treat dementia but the goal soon changed to the discovery of agents that might limit the consequences of having a stroke or offer neuroprotection as well as limit the associated decline in memory (Healy 2005). As a result, many drug companies have now turned their attention towards the development of these drugs. Memantine, galantamine, rivastigmine and donepezil are the medications developed for this purpose (Sadavoy 2007, Healy 2005) (see Ch 3 for more detail on these medications).

MANAGEMENT OF POLYPHARMACY IN THE OLDER PERSON

Polypharmacy also represents a difficult management problem for the older person and can lead to serious consequences (see Clinical alert 7.6). The special characteristics of older persons make them more vulnerable to problems related to polypharmacy. For example, symptoms of disease and age complicate medical and psychiatric treatment. Older persons are more likely to have multiple co-morbidities that require the use of multiple medications, which puts them at greater risk of drug interactions and side effect development. Therefore, where possible, polypharmacy with the older person should be avoided (see Clinical alert 7.7).

CLINICAL ALERT 7.6 – RISKS ASSOCIATED WITH POLYPHARMACY IN THE OLDER PERSON

- Greater likelihood of falls
- Greater difficulty in adequately diagnosing mental illness
- Adverse medication reactions, especially if dosage not reduced
- Greater likelihood of interactions

CLINICAL ALERT 7.7 – GUIDELINES FOR POLYPHARMACY IN THE OLDER PERSON

- Start low and go slow
- Monitor for signs of improvement and titrate dose accordingly
- Assess regularly for adverse signs
- Educate about medication side effects and management strategies
- Include consumer (wherever possible), carer and family in decisions

---

THE ETHICAL ISSUES ASSOCIATED WITH THE USE OF PSYCHOTROPIC MEDICATIONS IN OLDER PERSONS

Ethical issues have been raised about the use of psychotropic medications with older persons. The increasing use of psychotropic medications in this group is of particular concern given their enhanced susceptibility to drug side effects and other associated consequences of the treatment, such as falls and accidents. Further, the increasing use of benzodiazepines in older persons is alarming given that they are not recommended for first-line therapy with older people. Issues such as prescription and administration of psychotropic medications merely for the purpose of aiding the management of the older person with mental health problems have been mentioned. Concerns have also been raised about the ethics of prescribing and marketing memory enhancers to the elderly and the possible associated expectations for recovery that the family could develop. However, any improvement in cognitive functioning and quality of life, even if temporary, is considered to be justified by some in the area (Sadavoy 2007).

THE USE OF PSYCHOTROPIC MEDICATIONS IN INDIGENOUS PEOPLES

Mental health disorders are widespread among Indigenous Australian men and women who are hospitalised for mental and behavioural problems at 2.0 and 1.5 times the rate, respectively, of non-Indigenous Australians. Suicide among Indigenous Australians has increased over the past three decades to an alarming level. Between 1999 and 2001 the rate of suicide among Indigenous Australians in Queensland was 56% higher than the whole state with the rate for young men aged between 15 and 24 years 3.5 times higher. Approximately 83% of Indigenous Australians who committed suicide were aged less than 35 years, with most of the deaths by hanging. An emerging trend of child suicide has arisen in the last decade and, between 2004 and 2006, the six Aboriginal child suicides represented 20% of all such deaths in Queensland, whereas Indigenous Australians only make up 6.3% of the population (Hunter 2007). Surveys of Indigenous Australians have identified high rates of depression (McKendrick & Charles 2001) and other psychiatric disorders. Factors such as poverty, racism and dislocation from land and family are thought to be related to these findings. Indigenous Australians are more likely to live in rural and remote areas and thus experience a lack of access to appropriate services, including specialist services, which is recognised as problematic in those areas. It has also been proposed that access to and the use of health services are influenced by factors such as language skills, the availability of interpreters, concepts of health and illness, cultural factors, gender issues, physical set-up of services and method of delivery, the sensitivity of staff to Indigenous issues, the presence of appropriate Indigenous staff, racism, community ownership of services and confidentiality (Carson & Bailie 2004). A recent Australian study (Eley et al 2007) reported that Indigenous participants identified racism, shame, embarrassment and guilt as reasons that stopped them from accessing mental health services. The participants also revealed that they had limited understanding of mental health services or disorders so it is not surprising that they are reluctant to ask for help, especially when a lack of understanding is combined with the stigma of being labelled 'womba' or mentally ill.

Māori people have poorer health when compared to non-Māori people and this includes mental health. A study of Māori people accessing GP clinics found that they were more likely to present with diagnosable anxiety and depressive and substance use disorders (The MaGPIe Research

Group 2005). Pacific Island Nations people living in New Zealand are also known to experience higher rates of mental disorder and New Zealand-born Pacific Island Nations people experience significantly higher rates of mental disorder than Island-born Pacific people. In particular, they have a higher prevalence of suicidal ideation, suicide plans and suicide attempts than the general population and underutilise health services. These issues are more prevalent in the younger age group (Foliaki et al 2006). An audit of antipsychotic usage in the three health sectors of Auckland found significant differences in prescribing practices. The South Auckland region, where there are high numbers of Māori and Pacific Island Nations people, had higher rates of prescription of depot antispychotics, with flupenthixol the most commonly prescribed (40.4%), and people in this region were more likely to be prescribed higher doses of antipsychotics than people in the other, more affluent regions (Humberstone et al 2004).

Indigenous peoples tend to have different views about health and health care, mental disorder and treatment. They tend to lack knowledge of psychiatric nomenclature and currently accepted treatment methods and often report difficulty reading information or communicating in English. Of concern is the mental health staff attitude towards Indigenous people that suggests a heightened tendency to pathologise the behaviour of Indigenous, in particular 'black', people when compared to non-Indigenous people (Miranda et al 2002).

We also know that people from different races react differently to psychotropic medications. This is an important consideration when working with people from different cultural backgrounds who are prescribed psychotropic medications. Indigenous peoples of various countries also react differently to time and time-related events than their non-Indigenous counterparts. This has implications for the management of adherence with psychotropic medications in Indigenous populations. To date, little research has been conducted into the particular issue of psychotropic medication and Indigenous people. A recent Australian study (Usher et al 2007) found that mental health nurses perceived Indigenous inpatients as more likely to be prescribed and administered psychotropic medications, particularly PRNs or 'as needed' medications (to be discussed in detail in Ch 8). However, the small quantitative phase of that study indicated that, while Indigenous inpatients were prescribed higher rates of PRNs, they were actually administered less than their non-Indigenous counterparts. Indigenous Australians have also been found to experience difficulty managing their psychotropic medications, particularly in relation to issues of storage, maintenance of a medication regimen, feelings about taking the medications, sharing of prescriptions and medications and side effects (Kowanko et al 2004).

CONCLUSIONS

This chapter has provided an overview of the key issues regarding the use of psychotropic medications in special populations. The importance of being aware of the best available medication, correct dosages and special precautions has been outlined. References to a number of key articles have been provided for further reading if you wish to pursue some of the issues raised here in more detail, especially as they relate to your particular role in clinical practice.

Useful websites

National Prescribing Service (NPS) – providing useful information on all medications for health professionals and consumers, http://www.nps.org.au

Teratology Information Services (OTIS) – helping to prevent birth defects through education and research, http://www.otispregnancy.org/

The Massachusetts General Hospital Center for Women's Mental Health – providing current research outcomes of relevance to psychotropic medication and pregnant or breastfeeding women, http://www.womensmentalhealth.org/topics/breastfeeding.html

The New Zealand Mental Health Foundation – providing information on consumer perspectives, http://www.mhc.org.nz

Recommended reading

Hunter E 2007 Disadvantage and discontent: A review of issues relevant to the mental health of rural and remote Indigenous Australians. Australian Journal of Rural Health 15:88–93

McCauley-Elsom K, Kulkarni J 2007 Managing psychosis in pregnancy. The Royal Australian and New Zealand College of Psychiatrists 41:289–292

Miranda J, Lawson W, Escobar J 2002 Ethnic minorities. Mental Health Services Research 4(4):231–237

The MaGPIe Research Group, University of Otago at Wellington School of Medicine and Health Services, New Zealand 2005 Mental Disorders among Maori attending their general practitioner. Australian and New Zealand Journal of Psychiatry 39:401–406

Tiffin P A 2007 Managing psychotic illness in young people: A practical overview. Child and Adolescent Mental Health 12(4):173–186

Teaching and learning activities

- Outline the health professionals who may be involved in the care of a pregnant woman with a pre-existing mental illness who requires treatment with psychotropic medications. Consider the role each may play in ensuring the safest possible outcome for both the mother and baby. Also outline how collaboration between the team members might be facilitated.

- Many ethical issues have been raised regarding the use of psychotropic medication with young children. Some of these have been outlined in this chapter. Discuss this issue with friends and family and write an outline of the issues raised and the basis for the arguments made.
- Read the article by Miranda, Lawson and Escobar (2002) and outline the key issues involved in the development of negative attitudes to Indigenous people. Why do you think health professionals might pathologise the behaviour of Indigenous people and how might that interfere with consumer care?

References

Alanen H-A, Finne-Soveri H, Noro A et al 2006 Use of antipsychotic medications among elderly residents in long-term institutional care: A three-year follow-up. International Journal of Geriatric Psychiatry 21:288–295

Bolfek A, Jankowski J J, Waslick B et al 2006 Adolescent psychopharmacology: Drugs for mood disorders. Adolescent Med 17:789–808

Cabral P 2006 Attention deficit disorders: are we barking up the wrong tree? European Journal of Paediatric Neurology 10:66–77

Carson B E, Bailie R S 2004 National health workforce in discrete Indigenous communities. Australian and New Zealand Journal of Public Health 28(3):235–245

Eley D, Young L, Hunter K et al 2007 Perceptions of mental health service delivery among staff and Indigenous consumers: It's still about communication. Australasian Psychiatry 15(2):130–134

Empereur F, Baumann M, Briancon S 2003 Factors associated with the consumption of psychotropic drugs in a cohort of men and women aged 50 years and over. Journal of Clinical Pharmacy and Therapeutics 28:61–68

Ernst C, Goldberg J 2002 The reproductive safety profile of mood stabilizers, atypical antipsychotics, and broad-spectrum psychotropics. Journal of Clinical Psychiatry 63(4):42–55

Faraone S V 2004 Genetics of adult attention-deficit/hyperactivity disorder. Psychiatr Clin North Am 27:303–321

Faraone S V, Sergeant J, Gillberg C et al 2003 The worldwide prevalence of ADHD: Is it an American condition? World Psychiatry 2:104–113

Faraone S V, Perlis R H, Doyle A E et al 2005 Molecular genetics of attention deficit hyperactive disorder. Biological Psychiatry 57:1313–1323

Foliaki S A, Kokava J, Schaaf D et al for the New Zealand Mental Health Survey Research Team 2006 Twelve-month and lifetime prevalences of mental disorders and treatment contact among Pacific people in Te Rau Hinengaro: The New Zealand Mental health Survey. Australia and New Zealand Journal of Psychiatry 40:924–934

Greydanus D E, Pratt H D, Patel D R 2007 Attention deficit hyperactivity disorder across the lifespan: The child, adolescent, and adult. Dis Mon 53:70–131

Grover S, Avasthi A, Sharma Y 2006 Psychotropics in pregnancy: Weighing the risks. Indian Journal of Medical Research 123:497–512

Hale T W 2004 Medications and mothers' milk, 11th edn. Pharmasoft, Amarillo, TX

Hammerness P G, Vivas Fe M, Geller D A 2006 Selective serotonin reuptake inhibitors in pediatric psychopharmacology: A review of the evidence. Journal of Pediatrics 148:158–165

Hamrin V, Pachler M 2007 Pediatric bipolar disorder: Evidence-based psychopharmacological treatments. JCAPN 20(1):40–58

Harrison-Woolrych M, Garcia-Quiroga J, Ashton J et al 2007 Safety and usage of atypical antispsychotic medicines in children. Drug Safety 30(7):569–579

Healy D 2005 Psychiatric Drugs Explained, 4th edn. Churchill Livingstone, Edinburgh

Hopwood M J 2007 Psychotropic medication use in older people. Journal of Pharmacy Practice and Research 37(2):153–156

Humberstone V, Wheeler A, Lambert T 2004 An audit of output: Antipsychotic usage in the three health sectors of Auckland. Australian and New Zealand Journal of Psychiatry 38:240–245

Hunter E 2007 Disadvantage and discontent: A review of issues relevant to the mental health of rural and remote Indigenous Australians. Australian Journal of Rural Health 15:88–93

Ilett K F, Hackett L P, Kristensen J H et al 2004 Transfer of risperidone and 9-hydroxyrisperidone into human milk. The Annals of Pharmacotherapy 38:273–276

Iqbal M M, Sobhan T, Ryals T 2002 Effects of commonly used benzodiazepines on the foetus, the neonate and the nursing infant. Psychiatric Services 53:39–49

Jain A E, Lacy T 2005 Psychotropic drugs in pregnancy and lactation. Journal of Psychiatric Practice 11(3):177–191

Jensen P, Buitelaar J, Pandina G J et al 2007 Management of psychiatric disorders in children and adolescents with atypical antispychotics. Eur Child Adolesc Psychiatry 16:104–120

Kales H C, Valenstein M D, Kim H M et al 2007 Mortality risk in patients with dementia treated with antipsychotics versus other psychiatric medications. The American Journal of Psychiatry 164(10):1568–1576

Kowanko I, de Crespigny C, Murray H et al 2004 Better medication management for Aboriginal people with mental health disorders: A survey of providers. Australian Journal of Rural Health 12:253–257

Lacramioara S, Arnold L E 2007 Ethical issues in child psychopharmacology research and practice: Emphasis on preschoolers. Psychopharmacology 191:15–26

Laita P, Cifuentes A, Doll A et al 2007 Antipsychotic-related abnormal involuntary movements and metabolic and endocrine side effects in children and adolescents. Journal of Child and Adolescent Psychopharmacology 17(4):487–501

Lakhan S E, Hagger-Johnson G E 2007 The impact of prescribed psychotropics on youth. Clinical Practice and Epidemiology in Mental Health, 3(21). Available: http://www.cpementalhealth.com/content/3/1/21 20 Mar 2008

McCauley-Elsom K, Kulkarni J 2007 Managing psychosis in pregnancy. The Royal Australian and New Zealand College of Psychiatrists 41:289–292

McKendrick J, Charles S 2001 The Report of the Rumbalara Mental Health Project (vol 1). Department of Psychiatry, University of Melbourne, Melbourne

Malone K, Papagni K, Ramini S et al 2004 Antidepressants, antipsychotics, benzodiazepines, and the breastfeeding dyad. Perspectives in Psychiatric Care 40(2):73–86

Malone M, Ryan D O, Carnahan M et al 2007 Antipsychotic medication use in the elderly patient. Journal of Pharmacy Practice 20(4):318–326

Miranda J, Lawson W, Escobar J 2002 Ethnic minorities. Mental Health Services Research 4(4):231–237

Oates M 2003 Perinatal psychiatric disorders: A leading cause of maternal morbidity and mortality. British Medical Bulletin 67:219–229

Payne J L 2007 Antidepressant use in the postpartum period: Practical considerations. American Journal of Psychiatry 164:1329–1332

Perlis R H, Perlis C S, Wu Y et al 2005 Industry sponsorship and financial conflict of interest in the reporting of clinical trials in psychiatry. The American Journal of Psychiatry 162(10):1957–1960

Sadavoy J 2007 Psychopharmacology in the elderly: Successes, pitfalls, and precautions. Psychiatric Times 24(8):72–85

Shupikai Rinomhota A, Marshall P 2000 Biological aspects of mental health nursing. Churchill Livingstone, London

Solyom A E, Moreno J D 2005 Protection of children and adolescents in psychiatric research: An unfinished business. Healthcare Ethics Committee Forum 17:210–226

Spencer T J, Biederman J, Mick E 2007 Attention-deficit/hyperactivity disorder: Diagnosis, lifespan, comorbidities, and neurobiology. Journal of Pediatric Psychology 32:631–642

Stowe Z N 2007 The use of mood stabilizers during breastfeeding. Journal of Clinical Psychiatry 68(Suppl 9):22–28

Sved Williams A 2007 Antidepressants in pregnancy and breastfeeding. Australian Prescriber 30(5):125–127

The MaGPIe Research Group, University of Otago at Wellington School of Medicine and Health Services, New Zealand 2005 Mental Disorders among Maori attending their general practitioner. Australian and New Zealand Journal of Psychiatry 39:401–406

Tiffin P A 2007 Managing psychotic illness in young people: A practical overview. Child and Adolescent Mental Health 12(4):173–186

Trixler M, Tenyi T 1997 Antipsychotic use in pregnancy. Drug Safety 16(6):403–410

Usher K, Foster K, McNamara P 2005 Antipsychotic drugs and pregnant and breastfeeding women: The issues for mental health nurses. Journal of Psychiatric and Mental Health Nursing 12:713–718

Usher K, Foster K 2006 The use of psychotropic medications with breastfeeding women: Applying the available evidence. Contemporary Nurse 21(1):94–102

Usher K, Holmes C, Baker J et al 2007 Enhancing the understanding of clinical decision making for PRN medications within mental health facilities. Final report to the Queensland Nursing Council (QNC). School of Nursing, Midwifery and Nutrition, James Cook University, Brisbane, Qld

Viguera A C, Cohen L S 1998 The course and management of bipolar disorder during pregnancy. Psychopharmacology Bulletin 34:339–353

Viguera A C, Newport D J, Ritchie J et al 2007 Lithium in breast milk and nursing infants: clinical implications. The American Journal of Psychiatry 164(2):342–345

Ward S, Wisner K L 2007 Collaborative management of women with bipolar disorder during pregnancy and postpartum: pharmacologic considerations. Journal of Midwifery and Women's Health 52(1):3–13

Way C M 2007 Safety of the newer antidepressants in pregnancy. Pharmacotherapy 27(4):546–552

Webb R T, Howard L, Abel K M 2004 Antipsychotic drugs for non-affective psychosis during pregnancy and postpartum (Cochrane Review). John Wiley & Sons, Ltd. Available: http://www.update-software.com/abstracts/ab004411.htm 29 Jan 2007

Winans E 2001 Antipsychotics and breastfeeding. Journal of Human Lactation 17(4):344–347

Windle A, Elliot E, Duszynski K et al 2007 Benzodiazepine prescribing in elderly Australian general practice patients. Australia and New Zealand Journal of Public Health 31(4):379–381

Yaeger D, Smith H G, Altshuler L L 2006 Atypical antipsychotics in the treatment of schizophrenia during pregnancy and the postpartum. American Journal of Psychiatry 163(12):2064–2070

CHAPTER 8

SPECIAL ISSUES WITH THE USE OF PSYCHOTROPIC MEDICATIONS

Objectives

The information in this chapter will assist you to:

» Outline the key issues related to the use of psychotropic medications in behavioural management

» Understand the use of PRN or 'as needed' psychotropic medications and the related issues

» Describe the key issues involved in medication adherence

» Describe the impact of side effects such as metabolic syndrome and sexual dysfunction on the consumer

» Outline some of the main administration issues related to psychotropic medications including depot injections and polypharmacy

Key terms and abbreviations

Adherence
Euthymia
Non-adherence
Polypharmacy
Rapid tranquillisation
5-HT$_{1A}$ receptor – serotonin sub-type receptor 1A
BMI – body mass index
FGA – first generation antipsychotic

IMI – intramuscular injection
IVI – intravenous injection
MetS – metabolic syndrome
NMS – neuroleptic malignant syndrome
PRN – pro re nata or as needed
SD – sexual dysfunction
SGA – second generation antipsychotic

INTRODUCTION

This chapter covers some of the key issues that may arise with people prescribed and administered antipsychotic medications. We begin with the issues surrounding the use of psychotropic medications for the management of behavioural emergencies followed by an exploration of PRN or 'as needed' medications, a medication route often prescribed in inpatient settings. An important aspect related to psychotropic medication outcomes is addressed under the heading adherence. Further issues related to the use of psychotropic medications such as depot preparations and polypharmacy are then examined, followed by a discussion of potential side effects that can have a significant impact on the consumer, such as metabolic syndrome and sexual dysfunction.

BEHAVIOURAL EMERGENCIES AND THE USE OF PSYCHOTROPIC DRUGS

Agitation, a non-specific cluster of behaviours that is common in many psychiatric disorders, has the potential to readily escalate to aggression. This behaviour necessitates urgent intervention to reduce the likelihood of harm to the person and others in the environment. When managing these behaviours it is always preferable to use non-coercive treatments initially, such as de-escalation techniques (talk-down, clinical interview and environmental techniques). If these are ineffective or if the patient becomes combative, the implementation of more coercive interventions such as show of force, involuntary medication, physical restraint or seclusion may be required (Allen 2000). If psychotropic medication is selected as the best option available, the patient should be offered the choice of taking an oral medication initially. If this is refused, an intramuscular injection (IMI) is usually the next step. In situations where the oral medication is refused or where the behaviour is such that a rapid response is required, rapid tranquillisation with antipsychotics, benzodiazepines or other sedative drugs by IMI or intravenous injection (IVI) may be required (Rocca et al 2006). Rapid tranquillisation is the administration of a medication with the intent of calming or sedating an agitated or aggressive patient. The aim should always be to reduce patient distress, allow for improved communication and reduce the risks of injury to the patient and others (MacPherson et al 2005).

Evidence for the effectiveness of the pharmacological management of aggression is limited (refer to Table 8.1 for currently used options). The question of whether best clinical practice involves the use of first generation antipsychotics (FGAs) versus benzodiazepines versus a combination of both remains a topical issue. Meanwhile, the second generation antipsychotics (SGAs) have recently been introduced and, so far, there has been limited research undertaken to establish their effectiveness in the management of aggressive events (Yildiz et al 2003). FGAs used for the treatment of aggression include haloperidol and droperidol, found to be equally effective but with droperidol offering a more rapid effect coupled with a greater degree of sedation (Rocca et al 2006). Of the SGAs, oral risperidone (available as a dispersible oral dose) has been found to be equally as effective as haloperidol, and the new IMI formulations of olanzapine and ziprasidone now offer new treatment options for the management of aggressive incidents. Their broader efficacy and better safety profile, combined with the ease of transfer to oral maintenance after the initial episode, make them a better option than the FGAs (Yildiz et al 2003). Clozapine, an SGA, has been found to have a beneficial effect in reducing violence. Hence it has become a popular treatment option for forensic patients with a history of violence (Martin et al 2008). It is not, however, readily available in a parenteral form. Benzodiazepines such as clonazepam and midazolam are also popular choices for the management of aggressive and violent patients, either in combination with an FGA or on their own. Midazolam has been found to be more rapidly sedating than haloperidol (Rocca et al 2006). Care must be taken when using rapid tranquillisation, however, as serious drug interactions or over-sedation may result (see Clinical alert 8.1). Respiratory depression may occur with high doses of midazolam or droperidol, and cardiac arrhythmias with zuclopenthixol, so these medications must be used with caution. The patient must be closely observed following the administration of the medication and until full recovery has occurred.

TABLE 8.1 – PHARMACOLOGICAL OPTIONS FOR THE MANAGEMENT OF AGGRESSION

Drug class	Name	Preparation
First generation		
antipsychotic (FGA)	Haloperidol	Oral/IMI/IVI
	Droperidol	IMI
Second generation		
antipsychotic (SGA)	Risperidone	Oral wafer
	Olanzapine	Oral wafer/IMI/
	Ziprasidone	Oral/IMI
	Clozapine	
Benzodiazepine	Clonazepam	IMI
	Midazolam	IMI

CLINICAL ALERT 8.1 – PRECAUTIONS WHEN USING RAPID TRANQUILLISATION

Rapid tranquillisation may lead to over-sedation – a life threatening outcome. Patients receiving large doses of psychotropic medications, especially droperidol and midazolam, are at high risk of respiratory depression and must be carefully observed at all times. The common observations for an unconscious patient are recommended.

The use of involuntary medications with psychiatric inpatients is, however, a controversial management practice. An injectable medication is likely to be perceived as a threat, assault or punishment, making the establishment of a therapeutic alliance more difficult. Therefore, it is clinically prudent to offer an oral medication first. If an IMI or IVI medication must be used, the clinicians must act in a respectful and non-judgmental way when dealing with the patient to ensure they do not cause any further distress or embarrassment. Removing the patient's clothing and exposing their buttocks for an IMI medication is certainly an invasion of their privacy and has the potential to cause serious psychological consequences for the patient (MacPherson et al 2005). Hence, well experienced and trained staff, set procedures, briefing, debriefing and stress coping strategies are considered vital for the effective and safe management of agitated or aggressive inpatients (Rocca et al 2006) (see Thinking challenge 8.1).

Higher doses of psychotropics and polypharmacy are more commonly

---

THINKING CHALLENGE 8.1

Do you believe the need to reduce aggression and the risk of harm to others warrants the forcible administration of an injectable psychotropic medication? If yes, how can the potential for harm to the consumer be minimised? If no, how would you manage aggressive acts?

---

administered to aggressive patients. A recent study found an increased use of pro re nata (PRN) or as-needed psychotropic medication with aggressive patients, indicating they were generally more likely to receive a PRN than other patients. Continued administration of PRN psychotropic medications was also observed after an aggressive event (up to a further 36 hours), indicating the possibility that staff administered PRN in an attempt to reduce the likelihood of repeated aggressive episodes. The use of other somatic PRN medications was also increased during that period (Goedhard et al 2007). Further information of relevance to this section is contained below in relation to the prescription and administration of PRN psychotropic medications (see also Clinical alert 8.2).

CLINICAL ALERT 8.2 – PRECAUTIONS WITH PSYCHOTROPIC MEDICATION IN SPECIAL POPULATIONS

Special care must be taken when considering the choice and dosage of psychotropic medication for the management of aggression in the elderly, pregnant women and children.

These groups are vulnerable with regard to psychotropic medication for different reasons; therefore, they should not be exposed to the high levels that may be prescribed and administered during stressful situations.

PRN (PRO RE NATA OR AS-NEEDED) PSYCHOTROPIC ADMINISTRATION

The existing PRN system enables nurses to respond efficiently to a consumer's request to reduce agitation or distress or to respond rapidly to an aggressive event without the need to call the treating medical officer. It allows for a PRN medication to be administered at the request of the consumer or at the discretion of the nurse (Davies et al 2007). A common practice in psychiatric settings, especially in high dependency or intensive care units, the prescription and administration of PRN psychotropic medications is a frequently used adjunct to routine medications. Originally considered a viable alternative to restraint, it is now condemned by some as having merely replaced a physical restraint with a chemical one (Donat 2005). It has been suggested that, rather than being an independent decision of doctors, PRN prescription is the result of interactive dynamics between doctors and nurses (Craven et al 1987) where the nurses pressure the doctor to prescribe a wide range of medications available for PRN administration. Concerns have also recently been raised about PRN psychotropic medications being used as a 'quick fix' for the convenience of the organisation rather than for the benefit of the consumer (Davies et al 2007) and that they have become the primary intervention within acute care settings. Unfortunately, a recent study of inpatient charts indicated that alternative therapeutic interventions, such as de-escalation, talking or separating from the group, were not implemented as a first choice or even after the PRN event to prevent the need for further medication (Curtis et al 2007). Ideally, PRN psychotropic medication should only be implemented when alternative interventions have failed or the level of distress is so great that it is warranted. Alternatives to PRN psychotropic medication have, in fact, been trialled and found to be effective. A nurse-led activity-based intervention comprising of movement and games in the morning and relaxation sessions in the afternoon was shown to be successful in reducing the number of PRN medications administered in a psychiatric high dependency unit (Thomas et al 2006).

In general, antipsychotic medications and benzodiazepines are the main classes of medications prescribed for psychotropic PRN; however, antihistamines, anticholinergics, antimuscarinics and sedatives may also be prescribed and administered by this means. Internationally, within mental health settings, PRN medications have been reported to be prescribed to approximately 70–80% of consumers and administered to about 50% depending on the setting (Craven et al 1987, Thapa et al 2003, Geffen et al 2002, Dean et al 2006). Dean, McDermott and Marshall (2006) reported that almost three-quarters of a recent Australian sample were prescribed a

PRN medication during their inpatient stay and approximately half were administered at least one dose of the medication. Another Australian study reported that 73.4% of their sample received a PRN on at least one occasion during the month of data collection (Curtis et al 2007). These findings are similar to the findings from earlier studies.

Psychotropic PRN medication is usually administered orally or by IMI and, although prescribed by a doctor, is a commonly administered nursing intervention. Usually given in the first few days after admission and most frequently during the evening shift, especially from 6 pm onwards, PRN medications are also frequently administered at weekends (Usher et al 2001). Peaks in PRN administration tend to coincide with regular medication administration and meal times (Gray et al 1996, Stratton-Powell 2001). Reasons given for administering a PRN medication include agitation, threatening behaviour, irritability, abusiveness, insomnia, disruptiveness, assault and at the request of the consumer (Usher et al 2001). Environmental influences have also been suggested as relevant to the administration of PRN psychotropic medications. The study by Usher, Holmes, Baker and Stocks (2007) proposed that the physical and psychological environment in which the consumers were cared for had an effect on the individual's sense of security. Research has previously implicated the environment as a major factor in the creation of agitation and, hence, as an instigator of the need for PRN psychotropic medication. For example, consumers recently identified factors such as how the ward looks as well as feelings of safety and privacy as impacting on their sense of wellbeing within inpatient facilities (Brimblecombe et al 2007, Happell 2008). These factors may adversely affect a consumer's mental health and indirectly lead to an increase in anxiety, agitation and frustration, and ultimately aggression, which in turn impacts on the need for staff to resort to administering a PRN medication.

The demographics of those who receive psychotropic PRN medications within inpatient settings are interesting. Although insufficient research has been conducted to confirm gender as a correlate of PRN administration, early studies do suggest that males are more likely than females to receive PRN psychotropic medication (Curtis & Capp 2003, Usher et al 2001). Similarly, Craven and colleagues (1987) reported age as a correlate, finding that consumers aged 50 or older were associated with more PRN prescriptions in total, and specifically the prescription and administration of more sedatives/hypnotics. Ethnic difference has also been found to be a predictor of PRN prescription and administration. Recent studies by Gudjonsson et al (2000) and Hales and Gudjonsson (2004) found that black American inpatients were more likely than white inpatients to be administered a PRN psychotropic medication. However they noted that many confounding variables, including the over representation of black patients within secure units, may have accounted for those findings. A recent Australian study found that, while nurses believed the Indigenous patients in the unit were administered a greater number of PRN medications, this was in fact not true. Interestingly, the study found that, while Indigenous inpatients were prescribed psychotropic PRN medications at a higher rate than non-Indigenous inpatients, the data revealed they were actually administered PRN medications less often than the non-Indigenous inpatients (Usher et al 2007). Alarmingly, this may indicate that mental health professionals are more likley to pathologise the behaviour of certain ethnic groups of people (Miranda et al 2002), including members of different Indigenous groups.

Despite the importance placed on the use of PRN medications within inpatient settings, little research has been undertaken to establish the clinical effectiveness of the intervention. In fact, it has been suggested that, in the past, the use of PRN psychotropic medications has been primarily based on clinical experience and habit rather than evidence (Whicher et al 2003) and has in many cases contributed to adverse reactions or excess sedation (Geffen et al 2002). The decision-making processes involved in the prescription and administration of PRN psychotropic medications are complex. Frequently, prescriptions include several medications and offer a dose range (for example 50–100 mg of a specific medication) from which the clinician must choose. Thus, even though they are prescribed by doctors, nurses are the ones most often charged with the responsibility of administering these medications and therefore have an important role to play in assessing the need for, and making the appropriate decisions around, administering psychotropic PRN medications (Usher et al 2003).

A recent study by Baker et al (2007a) in the UK has gone some way to unravelling the decision making that nurses engage in when faced with the administration of a PRN psychotropic medication. They found that nurses' decisions to adminster the medications were influenced by safety, knowledge of the patient and levels of patient distress. They also found that nurses used PRN medication as a first rather than a last resort due to limited skills, fewer years of clinical experience, time pressures and low or inadequate staffing levels. The nurses in the study reported regularly using PRN medications as a first resort without any attempt to implement an alternative. A similar study conducted in Australia (Usher et al 2006b) found, in contrast, that nurses reported using alternatives to medication in many cases. However, some of the respondents in that study indicated that PRN medications were also used as an easy option for managing the ward. Even when nurses indicate that they have used alternatives to a PRN medication initially, there is little evidence to back this up in client inpatient files (Curtis et al 2007). Other factors that influenced the nurses' decisions to administer a PRN psychotropic medication include the mental state of the patient, for example whether they assessed the person as being psychotic or agitated, and staffing levels, such as the lack of experienced staff or high levels of casuals on the ward (Usher et al 2007).

Perhaps the most serious problems associated with psychotropic PRN administration are the risks of severe side effects, pharmacokinetic drug interactions, higher than recommended drug doses and abuse by uninformed mental health staff (Ayd 1985, Bowden 1999). A recent study found that as many as one-fifth of reviewed consumer inpatient records contained prescriptions for drug combinations that were judged to have the potential to cause serious interactions (Davies et al 2007). This is alarming given that these potential interactions could be fatal. In many instances, large doses of antipsychotics can result in debilitating, potentially fatal side effects such as tardive dyskinesia, akathisia and parkinsonism. In a worst case scenario, a patient could display a side effect such as akathisia (restlessness, inner tension, emotional unease), which could be confused with a psychiatric problem; as a result, the patient may be given additional doses of antipsychotic agents that will only worsen the patient's symptoms and lead to further hospitalisation. In situations such as these a large amount of responsibility is placed on the health professional, who must be able to distinguish between side effects and disturbances that are psychiatric in origin, and determine whether the combination of medications could have serious consequences for the consumer. This is even more of a concern when many PRN administrations occur during a time of emergency.

In the past, the drugs most often prescribed for PRN administration have been the FGAs, in particular drugs like haloperidol. There is now evidence to suggest that the benzodiazepines are just as effective as the FGAs in managing acute agitation and disturbed behaviour and should be the drug of choice when a PRN is considered the appropriate management of an adverse event or a distressed patient (Geffen et al 2002). The unwanted side effects of the antipsychotics, the FGAs in particular, make the benzodiazepine group the better alternative as these are generally better tolerated (Usher & Luck 2004). If an antipsychotic is to be prescribed, the SGAs, especially risperidone, ziprasidone and olanzapine, are considered the most effective for the purpose (Yildiz et al 2003). However, examination of current practice indicates that the FGAs continue to be used predominantly for PRN management of psychotic disturbance (Geffen et al 2002, Curtis et al 2007). This is a concern given the current information indicating this is not the best clinical option (see Thinking challenge 8.2). Wherever possible, PRNs should be administered at the lowest dose to avoid untoward side effects and, if needed, increased later. Best practice guidelines for the administration of PRN psychotropics were developed in the UK with the assistance of a panel of experts. They revealed four key themes: (i) service users should be more involved in all processes associated with PRN psychotropic medications; (ii) PRN medication must be administered for the purpose for which it was prescribed; (iii) prescriptions must be time limited, which encourages review; (iv) staff need to develop knowledge and awareness about potential side effects prior to administering them (Baker et al 2007b). See also Table 8.2 for a summary of decisions to be made when administering PRN psychotropic

THINKING CHALLENGE 8.2

Why do you think clinicians continue to prescribe and administer the FGAs when the evidence indicates that better alternatives are available? List some of the issues involved in this problem.

TABLE 8.2 – DECISIONS TO BE MADE REGARDING THE ADMINISTRATION OF PRN PSYCHOTROPIC MEDICATIONS

The first decision: when to give	To relieve agitation and psychotic symptoms when other alternatives have failed
The second decision: what to give	Whenever possible a benzodiazepine should be chosen but if antipsychotics are preferred then the SGAs are a better option
The third decision: how to give	Oral and IMI routes are effective. IMI are faster acting and should be chosen if the patient is aggressive or extremely distressed
The fourth decision: how much to give	Always give the lowest possible dose and administer a higher dose if needed again

(Adapted from Usher & Luck 2004)

medication.

To date, consumer perspectives relating to the prescription and administration of psychotropic PRNs have been poorly researched. Some studies have suggested that consumers sometimes request the administration of PRN medication (between 20% and 37% of the time) (Gray et al 1996, Usher et al 2001). However, other studies suggest that consumers would prefer being restrained or secluded in preference to receiving a PRN medication (Sheline & Nelson 1993). A recent qualitative study reported that consumers valued PRN medication, with 86% finding it useful or helpful. This finding related particularly to early on in inpatient treatment, for example the first few days after admission. However, the participants in that study also reported how they found the process surrounding PRN administration confusing and stigmatising, especially as they reported being provided with very little information about the PRN or whether there was in fact one prescribed for them. Refusal of PRN administration when requested by the consumer, however, has been reported to result in feelings of frustration, anger and embarrassment and, ultimately, in

CHAT BOX 8.1
Clearly the use of PRN medications in a mental health setting differs from their use in a general setting where they might be used for pain management. Why do you think they are perceived differently?

feelings of disempowerment (Baker et al 2006) (see Chat box 8.1).

THE PRESCRIPTION AND ADMINISTRATION OF DEPOT PREPARATIONS OF ANTIPSYCHOTIC DRUGS

Depot antipsychotic preparations, introduced in the 1960s, are a useful and well accepted method of managing situations where consumers experience difficulty with regularly taking their medication or are forgetful. In other words, they are used as a means of enhancing adherence with psychotropic medications. They are also helpful when the consumer is unable to take oral medications, or if intestinal absorption is questioned. In reality, however, the use of depot injections still requires some degree of willingness to take the medication on the part of the consumer. Some consumers like them as they suit their lifestyle while others find the need for regular injections uncomfortable.

Depot antipsychotics are long-acting, injectable forms of the drugs, produced by forming an ester from an alcohol group and a long chain fatty acid that is then dissolved in oil. This process increases the fat solubility 1000-fold (Masand & Sanjay 2003). When administered by deep IMI, the drug is de-esterified to release the active agent, which slowly diffuses into the circulation. The injections are usually given every 2 to 4 weeks (Therapeutic Guidelines 2003). When commencing this form of therapy it may also be necessary to supplement temporarily with an oral medication (Masand & Sanjay 2003).

Depot injections of antipsychotic medications must be used with caution in vulnerable groups. Few studies have been conducted on the safety of depot antipsychotics for the older person. Of the FGA medications, low doses of haloperidol and fluphenazine are the preferred depot antipsychotic for use with older persons as they tend to cause less sedation, postural hypotension and antimuscarinic effect. Of the SGAs, risperidone was the first to be approved as a long-acting injectable. To date it appears to have a favourable safety profile with the older person. Depot injections are unsuitable for use with pregnant and breastfeeding women in most cases and are not suitable for use with children and adolescents.

From the perspective of adherence to the medication regimen, it is important to remember that a well-targeted clinician–consumer relationship can help to promote medication adherence better than any other strategy (Marland et al 1999). In fact, it is considered the most important factor determining whether or not people continue to take their medications as prescribed. However, one study reported that the average time a nurse spent with a consumer during the administration of a depot antipsychotic injection was between 1 and 4 minutes (Muir-Cochrane 2001). A recent study of community mental health nurse attitudes towards depot injections found that 23% reported having little time for the consumer consultation, 34% believed depot injections to be an old-fashioned treatment modality and 44% considered them to be stigmatising (Patel et al 2005).

Knowledge of the consumer view on depot injections is extremely limited. One recent study reported how consumers appeared to benefit from attending the clinic to receive their regular injection, especially through regular contact and interaction with the community nurse (Phillips & McCann 2007). One consumer said:

> I feel I have enough time to raise anything, family things or whatever. Sometimes it's not necessary, but it's there if I need it.
>
> (Phillips & McCann 2007, p 581)

The consumer's right to be involved in choosing the route of administration of prescribed medications is just as important as their right to be involved in all other aspects of their care. Obviously consumers value the time made available to discuss their issues when visiting nurses for their depot injection, but they should also be involved in the original decision to have a depot prescribed rather than an alternative regular medication. Failure

BOX 8.1 – PSYCHOTROPIC MEDICATIONS AVAILABLE AS DEPOT INJECTIONS	
» Flupenthixol	» Haloperidol
» Fluphenazine	» Risperidone

to involve the consumer in these decisions can often worsen problems of adherence. See Box 8.1 for a list of psychotropic medications available as depot injections.

ADHERENCE AND NON-ADHERENCE WITH PSYCHOTROPIC DRUGS

Psychotropic medications have become the mainstay of treatment for most psychiatric disorders. However, even though most people describe gaining some benefits from taking the medications, many do not always take them reliably (Howland 2007). Adherence means taking a medication as it has been prescribed. The terms adherence and non-adherence now tend to be used in preference to the terms compliance and non-compliance, although basically they are interchangeable. Compliance tends to frame the issue in relation to the prescriber and administrator, whereas adherence is thought to recognise that the consumer also has a role to play in medication taking. Regardless, adherence to psychotropic drugs is recognised as a major impediment to effective drug treatment. If a medication is not taken as prescribed, the consumer's symptoms may not improve at the rate expected, leading the family and clinical team to suspect the medication is not working or is not as effective as it was originally. This can lead to unnecessary changes in treatment and poor outcomes for the consumer. On the other hand, adherence to prescribed medications can lead to improvement in the condition, facilitate the process of functional recovery and help prevent illness-related complications such as substance abuse and suicide (Howland 2007).

Adherence to medications of all types is an issue that is experienced across conditions to some degree. It is particularly problematic, however, for consumers with a mental disorder for whom ongoing adherence to a medication program is required. And it is especially problematic given the unpleasant and disabling effects of many of the antipsychotic medications, especially the traditional or FGA group. However, failure to take medications as prescribed is often the cause of relapse and readmission to hospital. In fact, adherence to the antipsychotic medication has been claimed as the single most important factor in deferring admission (Fernando et al 1990). Consumers with schizophrenia have significant issues where adherence to medication is concerned. The chronic nature of the illness and the stigmatisation associated with the disease, as well as the associated cognitive disturbance, poor insight and intolerable medication side effects, compound the problem (Singh et al 2006). Younger consumers, males and those living alone or without significant supportive relationships are also at higher risk of nonadherence to medications (Cooper et al 2007) (see Chat box 8.2). Thus, the issue of adherence is indeed complex as described below.

The reasons consumers give for not taking their psychotropic medications include but are not limited to: adverse side effects, especially in situations where the side effect impacts on the person's quality of life or

---

CHAT BOX 8.2

In a recent study one participant said:

My boys are the reason I take it. When the boys are here they say "Have you taken your medication, mum?"

(Usher et al 2006b)

This is a good example of how family and support persons are important in medication adherence.

---

where it may even cause more distress than the symptoms of the illness; insight about the illness and the importance of taking the prescribed medication regularly; lack of education about the medications and their expected adverse effects; the cost of the medications, especially when the consumer is prescribed more than one medication; and the complexity of the regimen (Usher et al 2001, Howland 2007). Against advice, however, some consumers stop taking their medications and, because they do not

---

CHAT BOX 8.3

A participant in a recent study outlined the issue of feeling well and, thus, not needing medication anymore:

Well I think I'm well and I think I don't need it (medication) anymore even though I can intellectualise that it is not true, and because of the side effects I think I'm well, I don't need to take it, I can get rid of these side effects, I could lose some weight ...

(Usher et al 2006b)

Nurses and other health professionals often find these statements difficult to respond to and, unfortunately, often resort to pressure to adhere to medication rather than trying to listen to the perspective of the consumer. Rather than force the issue of adherence, perhaps reinforcing progress and maintaining regular contact might be a better option with this person.

THINKING CHALLENGE 8.3

Think about your own situation. Have you or someone close to you ever had to take a medication for a long period? Outline some of the issues you faced or know that others close to you have experienced with long-term medication adherence.

---

relapse immediately, fail to see the connection between the medications and remaining well. Alternatively, when consumers are well they may falsely believe that they no longer require the prescribed medication (see Chat box 8.3 and Thinking challenge 8.3).

A number of strategies have been proposed to help overcome adherence issues. The method chosen may be dependent upon the cause of the consumer's non-adherence. Treatment-related interventions include use of oral disintegrating tablets or long-acting injections, dose reductions or switching medications, webster packs and prescribing medications that only require once daily doses (see Chat box 8.4). Disease-related interventions such as supportive therapy and psychoeducation therapy are also useful. Interventions that address psychological and social factors include: supportive groups; educating the consumer, family and friends about the medications; and developing supportive therapeutic alliances with the consumer (Singh et al 2006). The development of an effective therapeutic alliance is deemed the single most important factor in adherence improvement. This can be enhanced by regular contact with the consumer such as: visits, telephone calls or email contact; monitoring

---

CHAT BOX 8.4

A participant in a recent study described the strategy that helped them:

With that (webster packs), you can see a track record, if something does happen and you haven't had them at the right time, you know straight away. It is a big difference between taking them out of bottles, because it is like a bank book so to speak, keeping account of what you have, or don't have.

(Usher et al 2006b)

This quote demonstrates how what appears to be a simple strategy can have a significant outcome.

---

for signs of relapse; asking about concerns that arise from family, friends and the media related to the medications; and offering a non-judgmental approach (Howland 2007). Possibly the best approach is an intervention that includes a combination of those listed above.

As you will have recognised by now, the issue of medication adherence is complex and multifaceted (Happell et al 2002) and, unfortunately, rarely includes the perspective of the consumer (Happell et al 2004). Consumers who were asked why they did not take their medications as prescribed indicated they had forgotten or run out (37.4%), thought it was not needed (24.6%), had not wanted to take the medications (18.9%) due to the side effects (14.2%) and mentioned other issues such as concerns about combining the medication with alcohol (4.0%) (Cooper et al 2007). It is also possible that nonadherence is a deliberate act; that is, the consumer decides not to take the medication anymore for whatever reason or purposely avoids it for a period of time. For example, a consumer in a recent study said:

> I sleep too much with it (medication name), like tonight I'm not going to take any medication because I'm going to Brisbane early in the morning and

I don't want to miss my flight. So I won't take it tonight, I will probably take it tomorrow night.

(Usher et al 2006b)

Determining accurate methods of measuring adherence is challenging. Tablet counts, serum levels and self-reports are examples of measures that have been attempted. Most of these are, however, very subjective. Even the medication count is complicated as the person could take the pill from the bottle and dispose of it rather than take it. Even watching someone take their tablet is difficult and often misleading. This has made accurate measures and predictions of adherence difficult. Consumers have reported that, whenever they become ill, non-adherence is always suspected:

One of the first things they (nurses and doctors) assume is that a person isn't taking their medication, and it has been my experience with that, you're actually sick before you stop taking medication …

(Happell et al 2004, p 246)

SEXUAL DYSFUNCTION ASSOCIATED WITH THE USE OF PSYCHOTROPIC MEDICATIONS

All psychotropic medications may be associated with sexual dysfunction (SD) but the antipsychotics and antidepressants are the most likely to cause this side effect. The physiology of sexual function is interesting and complex. Primarily, and extremely simplistically, libido is mostly regulated by dopamine, sexual arousal by acetylcholine and nitric oxide and orgasm by serotonin and noradrenaline (Stimmel & Gutierrez 2006).

Antidepressant-induced SD is complex because it is difficult to determine whether the problem is caused by the illness or the medication. Further, while severe SD may be linked to antidepressant use in some people, it may also improve libido in others, depending upon the medications used. Among the antidepressants, those with the strongest serotonin effect exhibit the highest rates of SD. In particular, the SSRIs, while revolutionary in the treatment of depression, have a high incidence of sexual side effects. Rates of SD as high as 80% have been reported with SSRIs (Balon 2006) (refer to Box 8.2 for strategies to manage SD associated with SSRIs). In particular, the sexual side effects experienced with antidepressants include decreased libido, impaired erection, delayed or absent ejaculation and anorgasmia. These side effects are linked to relationship strain, quality of life and medication adherence (Stadler et al 2006) (see Chat box 8.5). It is important for the clinician to remember that delayed ejaculation and orgasm, symptoms most often associated with SSRIs, are not those most commonly associated with depression itself, whereas sexual desire is

---

BOX 8.2 – STRATEGIES FOR MANAGING SSRI-RELATED SEXUAL DYSFUNCTION (SD)

» Conduct a baseline assessment that includes sexual function prior to commencing the medication whenever possible
» Switch to a medication that has less associated SD
» Reduce dose of medication
» Suggest 'drug holidays' for short periods such as weekends

(Taken from Stadler et al 2006)

CHAT BOX 8.5

My husband became depressed 5 years ago and has been taking antidepressants ever since. He is much better now but still needs to take the pills. The worst part about that has been his problem with sex. It has made our relationship quite strained and difficult and doesn't look like getting any better soon.

This quote outlines the impact of the medication on the consumer and their relationship with their partner. It is always important to remember that partners and families are also impacted by these medications in some way.

(Balon 2006).

Erectile dysfunction (48%) and ejaculatory disturbance (45%) are prominent with antipsychotic medications. However, disturbances of libido, lubrication and orgasm can also occur. While the SGAs have a better side effect profile generally, some do have an impact on sexual function, and loss of libido and ejaculatory disorders have been reported (Stadler et al 2006).

Underreported cases of SD, especially by women, are thought to be high. Social and cultural factors impact on a person's willingness to discuss their SD and their willingness to seek help. In addition, these factors are also related to what a person will think is normal sexual function (Werneke et al 2006). Effective management of SD should include a baseline assessment as it is not sufficient to ask someone to remember a month later whether they had that problem initially. Switching medications, reduction in dosage or 'drug holidays' for short periods of time have all been suggested as useful strategies for the management of SD (Stadler et al 2006).

METABOLIC SYNDROME (MetS) AND ITS MANAGEMENT

Many psychotropic medications, including both FGAs and SGAs, antidepressants and mood stabilisers, are associated with metabolic disturbances, especially weight gain. However, the newer SGAs, while providing great relief from the symptoms of schizophrenia for many, are strongly linked to a number of serious side effects such as obesity, hyperlipidaemia, type 2 diabetes mellitus and diabetic ketoacidosis, which together make up what is known as metabolic syndrome (MetS) (Henderson et al 2005). (Refer to Table 8.3 for a list of SGAs linked to MetS.) The weight gain associated with SGAs usually occurs during the first 4–12 weeks of treatment. After the initial period the weight gain continues at a lower level or may even stabilise, except in the case of clozapine and olanzapine where the weight gain tends to continue over a prolonged period of time (Tschoner et al 2007). One recent Australian study of clozapine use in a forensic population, however, found an average weight increase of 6 kg after 12 months and 15 kg after 24 months (Martin et al 2008). The weight gain associated with SGAs is a concern given that people with schizophrenia are known to have a shorter life expectancy than the rest of the general population (perhaps as much as

TABLE 8.3 – SECOND GENERATION ANTISPYCHOTICS LINKED TO METABOLIC SYNDROME			
Atypical antipsychotic	Weight gain	Risk for diabetes	Dyslipidaemia
Clozapine	+++	+	+
Olanzapine	+++	+	+
Risperidone	++	+	IR
Quetiapine	++	IR	IR
Aripiprazole	+/–	–	–
Ziprasidone	+/–	–	–
Amisulpride	–	–	–
+: increasing effect; –: no effect; IR: inconclusive results			

(Adapted from Tschoner et al 2007, p 1357)

9–12 years) anyway. The evidence for a link between schizophrenia and diabetes is, however, not a new phenomenon as there has been interest in the link between antipsychotic medications, weight gain, diabetes and the potential for the development of MetS since the 1960s (Usher et al 2006a).

MetS is the development of a cluster of metabolic abnormalities associated with an increased risk of cardiovascular disease. It includes: weight gain, especially abdominal or visceral; diabetes; atherogenic lipid profile (increased low-density lipoprotein (LDL) cholesterol and triglyceride levels and reduced high-density lipoprotein (HDL) cholesterol); and elevated blood pressure (Antai-Otong 2004, Holt et al 2005). Unfortunately, these symptoms often go undetected or unreported in people with schizophrenia. Abdominal or visceral weight gain is highly associated with an increased risk of developing insulin resistance and/ or MetS and for type 2 diabetes mellitus. Diabetes mellitus is at almost epidemic proportions worldwide. The link between SGAs and the increased incidence of type 2 diabetes mellitus is thought to be caused by an increase in body weight or the direct effects of the antipsychotic agents on glucose transportation, elevation of serum leptin and antagonism of serotonin 1A (5-HT1$_A$) receptors decreasing pancreatic β-cell responsiveness (Citrome et al 2005).

Significant weight gain is the most noticeable sign of MetS. People with schizophrenia have been found to have a higher incidence of elevated body mass index (BMI) when compared to the general population, with a significantly higher proportion of females being overweight or obese when compared to other women. This increased weight can be explained in a number of ways, taking into account factors such as a more sedentary lifestyle, changes in habits of daily living as well as medication intake. The impact of weight gain associated with psychotropic medications is so serious, however, some consumers have reported stopping the medication because of the associated demoralisation and stigma. Weight gain is also linked to reduced quality of life and social retreat (Tschoner et al 2007). Diabetes is up to three times more prevalent in people taking both typical and atypical antipsychotics than in the general population. Clozapine is associated with a 1.4-fold higher prevalence than the FGAs, while olanzapine is associated with a 1.3-fold higher prevalence. The relative risk for developing diabetes appears to be lower with quetiapine and risperidone and neutral for the newer SGAs (Tschoner et al 2007).

The effective management of people taking antipsychotic medications is important to prevent the development of MetS. Weight gain should be regularly monitored as it is a major contributor to poor health outcomes. Switching to a medication with a better metabolic profile may also be considered depending on the individual response to the treatment. Early intervention, which should occur when the person begins taking the medication, should target reduced calorie intake and increased exercise as this has been shown to have a positive effect on weight gain (Tschoner et al 2007) (see Box 8.3).

POLYPHARMACY

Polypharmacy, or combination therapy, refers to the concurrent use

---

BOX 8.3 – STRATEGIES FOR MANAGING ANTIPSYCHOTIC MEDICATION-INDUCED WEIGHT GAIN

» Conduct a baseline assessment of weight, height, blood glucose and lipid levels
» Monitor regularly once commenced on medications
» Commence reduced calorie diet and increased exercise program early in treatment
» Educate consumer and partner/family/carer
» Consider switching medications if weight gain increases
» Include the consumer in all medication decisions

(Adapted from Usher et al 2006a, Tschoner et al 2007)

---

of multiple medications. It usually has a negative connotation because it appears to indicate that the concurrent use of the medications is inappropriate. Of course this may not always be the case. With regard to the use of psychotropic medications, however, polypharmacy has more serious implications. Here it usually means the use of two or more antipsychotics simultaneously, especially for the treatment of schizophrenia, with the goal of increasing the overall efficacy of the treatment (Masand et al 2006). While it is not considered an ideal practice, polypharmacy is common. Australian and American studies found that 13% of all outpatients with schizophrenia received more than one antipsychotic medication (Keks et al 1999, Tapp et al 2003). In the study by Keks et al (1999), 8% of subjects were on a combination of FGAs and SGAs, 5% were on FGAs and a depot and 3% were on oral FGAs. Other studies have reported rates of polypharmacy as high as between 11% and 25% (Masand et al 2006). Polypharmacy is not limited to antipsychotics, however. A recent survey of Australian doctors working in psychiatry reported that 79% had used combination antidepressants, most often an SSRI coupled with a tricyclic but also frequently the combination of mirtazapine and venlafaxine (Horgan et al 2007). Combinations of other psychotropic medications are also common.

Reasons given for polypharmacy with antipsychotic medications include concern over an initial poor response rate with an antipsychotic, the use of a combination while 'switching' to another medication, the combination of an FGA with an SGA when the FGA is used as the lead-in while the SGA takes effect, and where an FGA is used as a 'top up' for an SGA when symptoms worsen in order to prevent a full exacerbation of psychiatric symptoms (Tapp et al 2003). With regard to antidepressants, polypharmacy is used to treat non-responders and the combination of mirtazapine and venlafaxine in the USA is known as *'Californian rocket fuel'* (Horgan et al 2007).

The disadvantages associated with polypharmacy are serious. They include: the potential to experience more frequent or severe side effects, especially the more serious ones; the increased risk of developing toxicity; non-adherence; and a lack of understanding of the contribution of each agent towards any noticed improvement (Safer et al 2003). This is a major concern given that some of the side effects from psychotropic medications are irreversible and others potentially fatal.

The use of concomitant psychotropic medications, which has been a practice for some time, appears to be increasing. This suggests that clinical judgment sometimes overrides pharmacological guidelines even though there is no evidence to support the combination of psychotropic medications. Therefore, it is evident that further research is required to determine levels of safety and to propose guidelines for safe practice when polypharmacy is used.

CONCLUSIONS

This chapter covered a number of important issues related to psychotropic medications. It is important for clinicians to develop an awareness of the issues faced by consumers when they use psychotropic medications to better assist them to implement strategies to manage their lives more effectively. Some of the issues contained in this chapter are critical to successful consumer outcome and warrant further attention. We hope you have enjoyed this section of the book and recognise its importance to clinical practice.

Useful websites

Australian Mental Health Consumer Network – one of the peak consumer groups in Australia, http://amhcn.org.au/

The New Zealand Mental Health Foundation – peak consumer group in New Zealand, http://www.mhc.org.nz

Websites containing helpful information on MetS:

http://www.world-heart-federation.org/

http://www.idf.org/

Recommended reading

Allen M H 2000 Managing the agitated psychotic patient; a reappraisal of the evidence. Journal of Clinical Psychiatry 61(Suppl 14):S1–S20

Baker J, Lovell K, Easton K et al 2006 Service users' experiences of 'as needed' psychotropic medications in acute mental healthcare settings. Journal of Advanced Nursing 56(4):354–362

Rocca P, Villari V, Bogetto F 2006 Managing the aggressive and violent patient in the psychiatric emergency. Progress in Neuro-Psychopharmacology & Biological

Psychiatry 30:586–598

Usher K, Foster K, Park T 2006a The metabolic syndrome and schizophrenia: The latest evidence and nursing guidelines for management. Journal of Psychiatric and Mental Health Nursing 13:730–734

Teaching and learning activities

- Interview a clinician currently working in the area of psychiatry. Ask them to describe a recent aggressive situation they have managed and outline the techniques they used and how they established their effectiveness. After the interview, read some of the inpatient files and look for evidence of interventions used, including PRN psychotropic medications.

- Remember when you have been prescribed a long course of a medication. Try to think of some of the main obstacles you faced to taking the medication exactly as prescribed. Write these down and share with others in your class and read theirs. How were they different? Do you think you would experience difficulty taking a medication for a year or more? If yes, write down and share with your class mates.

- Outline the major side effects related to SGAs and also list some of the key issues for the consumers taking the medications and their families.

- Consider the impact of antidepressants on SD and how that has the potential to impact on the consumer's relationship. How would you advise a consumer experiencing this side effect who is still clinically depressed yet raises concerns for the future of their relationship?

References

Allen M H 2000 Managing the agitated psychotic patient; a reappraisal of the evidence. Journal of Clinical Psychiatry 61(Suppl 14):S1–S20

Antai-Otong D 2004 Metabolic effects associated with atypical antipsychotic medications. Perspectives in Psychiatric Care 40:70–72

Ayd F J 1985 Problems with orders for medication as needed. American Journal of Psychiatry 142:939–942

Baker J, Lovell K, Easton K et al 2006 Service users' experiences of 'as needed' psychotropic medications in acute mental healthcare settings. Journal of Advanced Nursing 56(4):354–362

Baker J, Lovell K, Harris N 2007a Mental health professionals' psychotropic pro re nata (prn) medication practices in acute inpatient mental health care: A qualitative study. General Hospital Psychiatry 29:163–168

Baker J, Lovell K, Harris N et al 2007b Multidisciplinary consensus of best practice for pro re nata (PRN) psychotropic medications within acute health settings: A Delphi study. Journal of Psychiatric and Mental Health Nursing 14:478–484

Balon R 2006 SSRI-associated sexual dysfunction. American Journal of Psychiatry 163(9):1504–1509

Bowden M F 1999 Audit: prescription of 'as required' (p.r.n.) medication in an inpatient setting. Psychiatric Bulletin 23:413–416

Brimblecombe N, Tingle A, Murrells T 2007 How mental health nursing can best improve service users' experiences and outcomes in inpatient settings: Responses to a national consultation. Journal of Psychiatric and Mental Health Nursing 14:503–509

Citrome L, Blonde L, Damatarca C 2005 Metabolic issues in patients with severe mental illness. Southern Medical Association 98(7):714–720

Cooper C, Bebbington P, King M et al 2007 Why people do not take their psychotropic drugs as prescribed: Results of the 2000 National Psychiatric Morbidity Survey. Acta Psychiatrica Scandinavica 116:47–53

Craven J, Voore P, Voineskos G 1987 PRN medication in psychiatric inpatients. Canadian Journal of Psychiatry 32:199–203

Curtis J, Capp K 2003 Administration of 'as needed' psychotropic medication: A retrospective study. Journal of Mental Health Nursing 12:229–234

Curtis J, Baker J, Reid A R 2007 Exploration of therapeutic interventions that accompany the administration of p.r.n. ('as required') psychotropic medication within acute mental health settings: A retrospective study. International Journal of Mental Health Nursing 16:318–326

Davies S J C, Lennard M S, Ghahramani P et al 2007 PRN prescribing in psychiatric inpatients – potential for pharmacokinetic drug interactions. Psychopharmacology 21(2):153–160

Dean A J, McDermott B M, Marshall R T 2006 Psychotropic medication utilization in a child and adolescent mental health service. Journal of Child and Adolescent Psychopharmacology 16(3):273–285

Donat D C 2005 Special section on seclusion and restraint: Encouraging alternative seclusion, restraint and reliance on p.r.n. drugs in a public psychiatric hospital. Psychiatric Services 56:1105–1108

Fernando M L, Velamoor V R, Cooper A J et al 1990 Some factors relating to satisfactory post-discharge community maintenance of chronic psychotic patients. Canadian Journal of Psychiatry 35:71–73

Geffen J, Sorensen L, Stokes J et al 2002 Pro re nata medication for psychoses: An audit of practice in two metropolitan hospitals. Australian and New Zealand Journal of Psychiatry 36:649–656

Goedhard L E, Stolker J J, Nijman H L I et al 2007 Aggression of psychiatric patients associated with the use of as-needed medications. Pharmacopsychiatry 40:25–29

Gray R J, Smedley N S, Thomas B L 1996 Administration of PRN medication by mental health nurses. British Journal of Nursing 5(21):1317–1322

Gudjonsson G, Rabe-Hesketh S, Wilson C 2000 Violent incidents on a medium secure unit: The target of assault and the management of incidents. The Journal of Forensic Psychiatry 11:105–118

Hales H, Gudjonsson G 2004 Effect of ethnic differences on the use of prn (as required) medication on an inner London Medium secure unit. Journal of

Forensic Psychiatry and Psychology 15(2):303–313

Happell B 2008 Determining the effectiveness of mental health services from a consumer perspective: Part 2: Barriers to recovery and principles for evaluation. International Journal of Mental Health Nursing 17:123–130

Happell B, Manias E, Pinikahana J 2002 The role of the inpatient mental health nurse in facilitating patient adherence to medication regimes. International Journal of Mental Health Nursing 11:251–259

Happell B, Manias E, Roper C 2004 Wanting to be heard: Mental health consumers' experiences of information about medication. International Journal of Mental Health Nursing 13(4):242–248

Henderson D C, Cagliero E, Copeland P M et al 2005 Glucose metabolism in patients with schizophrenia treated with atypical antipsychotic agents. Archives of General Psychiatry 62:19–28

Holt R I G, Peveler R C, Byrne C D 2005 Schizophrenia, the metabolic syndrome and diabetes. Diabetic Medicine 21(6):515–523

Horgan D, Dodd S, Berk M 2007 A survey of combination antidepressant use in Australia. Australasian Psychiatry 15(1):26–29

Howland R H 2007 Medication adherence. Journal of Psychosocial Nursing 45(9):15–18

Keks N A, Hope J, Krapivensky N et al 1999 Use of antipsychotics and adjunctive medications by an inner urban community psychiatric service. Australian and New Zealand Journal of Psychiatry 33:896–901

MacPherson R, Dix R, Morgan S 2005 A growing evidence base for management guidelines. Advances in Psychiatric Treatment 11:404–415

Marland G R, Sharkey V, Ward E 1999 Depot neuroleptics, schizophrenia and the role of the nurse: Is practice evidence based? Journal of Advanced Nursing 30(6):1255–1262

Martin A, O'Driscoll C, Samuels A 2008 Clozapine use in a forensic population in a New South Wales prison hospital. Australian and New Zealand Journal of Psychiatry 42:141–146

Masand P S, Sanjay S 2003 Long-acting injectable antipsychotics in the elderly: Guidelines for effective use. Drugs and Aging 20(15):1099–1110

Masand P S, Tharwani H M, Patkar A A 2006 Polypharmacy in schizophrenia. International Journal of Psychiatry in Clinical Practice 10(4):258–263

Miranda J, Lawson W, Escobar J 2002 Ethnic minorities. Mental Health Services Research 4(4):231–237

Muir-Cochrane E 2001 The case management practices of community mental health nurses: Doing the best we can. Australian and New Zealand Journal of Mental Health Nursing 10:210–220

Patel M X, DeZoysa N, Baker D et al 2005 Antipsychotic depot medication and attitudes of community psychiatric nurses. Journal of Psychiatric and Mental Health Nursing 12:237–244

Phillips L, McCann E 2007 The subjective experience of people who regularly receive depot neuroleptic medication in the community. Journal of Psychiatric and Mental Health Nursing 14:578–586

Rocca P, Villari V, Bogetto F 2006 Managing the aggressive and violent patient in the psychiatric emergency. Progress in Neuro-Psychopharmacology & Biological Psychiatry 30:586–598

Safer D J, Zito J M, dosReis S 2003 Concomitant psychotropic medication for youths. American Journal of Psychiatry 160(3):438–449

Sheline Y, Nelson T 1993 Patient choice: Deciding between psychotropic medication and physical restraints in an emergency. Bulletin of the American Academy of Psychiatry and Law 21(3):321–329

Singh A C, Massey A J, Thompson M D et al 2006 Addressing nonadherence in the schizophrenia population. Journal of Pharmacy Practice 19(6):361–368

Stadler T, Bader M, Uckert S et al 2006 Adverse effects of drug therapies on male and female sexual function. World Journal of Urology 24:623–629

Stimmel G L, Gutierrez M A 2006 Sexual dysfunction and psychotropic medications. CNS Spectrums 11(8) (Suppl 9):24–30

Stratton-Powell H 2001 PRN lorazepam: The nurse's judgement, the nurse's decision. In: The School of Nursing, Midwifery and Social Work, Vol. Master of Philosophy, The University of Manchester, Manchester

Tapp A, Wood A E, Secrest L et al 2003 Combination antipsychotic therapy in clinical practice. Psychiatric Services 54(1):55–59

Thapa P B, Shanna L P, Owen R R et al 2003 P.R.N. (as needed) orders and exposure of psychiatric inpatients to unnecessary psychotropic medications. Psychiatric Services 54:1282–1286

Therapeutic Guidelines: Psychotropics 2000 Therapeutic Guidelines Limited, North Melbourne, Australia

Thomas B, Jones M, Johns P et al 2006 P.r.n. medication use in a psychiatric high-dependency unit following the introduction of a nurse-led activity programme. International Journal of Mental Health Nursing 15:266–271

Tschoner A, Engl J, Laimer M et al 2007 Metabolic side effects of antipsychotic medication. International Journal of Clinical Practice 61(8):1356–1370

Usher K, Lindsay D, Sellen J 2001 Mental health nurses' PRN psychotropic medication administration practices. Journal of Psychiatric and Mental Health Nursing 8:383–390

Usher K, Holmes C, Lindsay D et al 2003 PRN psychotropic medications: The need for nursing research. Contemporary Nurse 14(3):248–257

Usher K, Luck L 2004 Psychotropic PRN: A model for best practice management of acute psychotic behavioural disturbance in inpatient psychiatric settings. International Journal of Mental Health Nursing 13:18–21

Usher K, Foster K, Park T 2006a The metabolic syndrome and schizophrenia: The latest evidence and nursing guidelines for management. Journal of Psychiatric and Mental Health Nursing 13:730–734

Usher K, Hay P, Quirk F et al 2006b Development of a questionnaire to measure antipsychotic medication compliance. Paper presented at the Australian and New Zealand College of Mental Health Nurses 32nd Annual International Conference, Alice Springs, NT, 4th October

Usher K, Holmes C, Baker J et al 2007 Enhancing the understanding of clinical decision making for PRN medications within mental health facilities. Final report to the Queensland Nursing Council (QNC). School of Nursing, Midwifery and Nutrition, James Cook University, Brisbane, Qld

Werneke U, Northey S, Bhugra D 2006 Antidepressants and sexual dysfunction. Acta Psychiatrica Scandinavica 114:384–397

Whicher E, Morrison M, Douglas-Hall P 2003 'As Required' Medication Regimes for Seriously Mentally Ill People in Hospital. The Cochrane Library, Oxford

Yildiz A, Sachs G S, Turgay A 2003 Pharmacological management of agitation in emergency. Emergency Medicine Journal 20:339–346. Available: http://www.emjonline.com 19 Nov 2007

INDEX

abuse *see* substance misuse
acamprosate 118
acetaldehyde 120
acetylcholine (ACh) 24, 25
acetylcholinesterase inhibitors
  adverse effects 59
  for Alzheimer's dementia 59
  for dementia 58, 62
  dosage 59
  pharmacodynamics 59
  prescribing issues 62
ADD *see* attention deficit disorder (ADD)
addiction 111
ADHD *see* attention deficit/hyperactivity
  disorder (ADHD)
adherence to psychotropic medications
  10, 171–2
  determining level of adherence 175
  strategies to overcome adherence issues
    173–4
  see also non-adherence to psychotropic
    medications
adolescents *see* children and adolescents
adrenergic muscarinic receptors,
  blocking of 76
adrenergic neurotransmission,
  alterations in anxiety disorders 98
adrenergic receptors, blocking of 45–6
affect
  major disturbances 68
  normal 67
affect disorders 67, 68
  antidepressants for 69, 71
  consumer perspectives 81–3
  pathophysiology 70–3
  psychotherapeutic counselling 69
  treatment strategies 69
aged care facilities, rates of use of
  psychotropic medications 149
aged persons *see* older persons
aggression
  medications for, in children and

adolescents 140
oral versus injectable medications 162,
  163–4
pharmacological management 162–3
psychotropic medications 162–6
somatic PRN medications 164
agitation
  environment as factor in 166
  medications for, in children and
    adolescents 140
  oral versus injectable medications 162,
    163–4
  psychotropic medications 162
agoraphobia 96
AIMS (Abnormal Involuntary Movement
  Scale) 46
akathisia 44
alcohol 112
  regional statistics on use 113
alcohol dependence
  drug treatment 118–20
  family and friends recognition of a
    person's dependence 123
  reasons for developing in men 123
alcohol use problems, in young people
  122
alcohol withdrawal 120
  features 117
Alcoholics Anonymous (AA) 114
aldehyde dehydrogenase 12
alprazolam 100, 133
altered brain structure, in schizophrenia
  41–2
Alzheimer's dementia
  amyloid plaques 56–7
  depression in 58
  genetic predisposition 57–8
  histological hallmarks 56–7
  medications for 151
  neurofibrillary tangles 56, 57
  pathophysiology 55–8
  pharmacology of drugs for 58–9

186

breast milk, transfer of psychotropic
medications to 136
breastfeeding
anticonvulsant use 137–8
antidepressant use 137
antipsychotics use 136
benzodiazepine use 138
depot antipsychotic preparation
unsuitability 171
lithium use 137
and mental disorders 135
psychotropic medication use 135–8
buprenorphine, for opioid withdrawal
120, 121
bupropion
for ADD/ADHD 147
adverse effects 137
for nicotine withdrawal 122
buspirone
adverse effects 102
for anxiety disorders 98, 102
butyrophenones, adverse effect profiles
46

'Californian rocket fuel' 179
cAMP response element binding protein
(CREB) 72, 117
cannabis 112
cannabis use
linked with mental health problems
113–14
prevalence 112
and psychosis 52
cannabis withdrawal, features 117
carbamazepine 85, 133, 138
carer perspectives
on dementia 59–62
clinicians sensitivity towards carers
61–2
psychological distress of carers 60–1
unmet needs in looking after loved
ones with dementia 61
on substance misuse 123
catecholamine neurotransmission 145,
147
caudate nucleus of basal ganglia
role in anxiety 96–8
role in automatic checking behaviours
98
cell membrane 23
central nervous system (CNS),
psychotropic drug entry into 28
central nervous system (CNS) stimulants

for ADD/ADHD 145–6
adverse effects 146
mechanisms of action at synapse 146
centrally acting dopamine receptor
antagonists see dopamine receptor
antagonists
cerebellum 22, 145
cerebral cortex 21
role in cognition and perception 38
cerebral dominance 22
cerebral hemispheres 21, 22
cerebrum 21
children and adolescents
antipsychotic use 139–41
medications
for agitation/aggression 140
for attention deficit disorders 144–7
for depression and bipolar disorder
141–4
psychotropic medications in 138–47
ethical issues 147–8
and sedating antihistamines 107
chlorpromazine 3, 4, 43
use during pregnancy 131–2
cholinergic nerve cell death, in
Alzheimer's dementia 55, 59, 60
cingulate gyrus 67, 73
citalopram 75, 137
classical antipsychotics see first
generation antipsychotics
clomipramine 76
clonazepam 133, 163
clonidine 147
clozapine 47
adverse effects in paediatric patients
140, 141
for aggression 162–3
in children and adolescents 140, 141
not recommended while breastfeeding
136
in pregnancy 132
risk of neutropenia 47
side effects 4, 47, 132
for treatment-resistant schizophrenia 47
weight gain associated with 141, 177
Clozapine Patient Monitoring System
guidelines 47
cocaine 112, 114
cognition 37
brain regions role in 38
disturbances of 37
factors involved 38
normal 37

cognition disorders
    chemical imbalances in
        neurotransmitter pathways 39
    clinical manifestations 39
    see also Alzheimer's dementia;
        psychosis; schizophrenia
cognitive behavioural therapy 94
    in anxiety management 93
    in management of sleep disturbances 94
community-based services 5–6
community-based treatment orders 8
community mental health services 6
Community Treatment Orders 8–9
complementary and alternative
    therapies, for depression 78–9, 83
compliance *see* adherence to
    psychotropic drugs
congenital malformations
    from anticonvulsants 133
    from antidepressants 133
    from benzodiazepines 133–4
    from lithium 132
    risk from psychotropic medications
        131, 132, 133–4
consultancy teams 6
consumer perspectives
    on antipsychotic medications 8, 9–10,
        51–3
    on anxiety and its treatment 102–3
    benefits/disadvantages of
        psychotropics 11
    on depot antipsychotics 53, 171
    on disturbances in mood and affect 81–3
    experiences of depression 81–3
    factors influencing recovery from
        depression 83
    loss of self-control when taking
        antipsychotics 52, 53
    on non-adherence to psychotropic
        medications 172–3, 174
    PRN psychotropic administration
        169–70
    side effects of psychotropic medications
        9, 13, 52, 53
    of stigma and discrimination due to
        mental health problems 5, 11, 81
    on substance misuse 122–3
continuing care 6
corpus callosum 21, 145
corpus striatum 145
    role in cognition and perception 38
creatine phosphokinase (CFK) levels
    50, 52

creatinine clearance 31
cyclothymia 67
    features and symptoms 68
cytochrome P450 (CYP) enzymes 29–31
    psychotropic drug interactions 29–30

D_1–D_5 receptors, distribution and
    function 43
D_2 receptor
    antipsychotic agents affinity for 43, 45
    moderation by 5-HT_2 receptors 47
DAI (Drug Attitude Inventory) 46
daytime sleepiness 105
deinstitutionalisation 5, 6
    failure of 7
deltaFosB 117
delusions 39
dementia
    Alzheimer's *see* Alzheimer's dementia
    antipsychotic prescribing rate 149
    carer perspective 59–62
    medications for 151
    prescribing and administration issues
        62
    types of 55
dependence *see* alcohol dependence;
    drug dependence
depot antipsychotic preparations
    cautions 170–1
    consumer perspectives 53, 171
    definition 170
    drug availability 171
    for older persons 170
    prescription and administration 170–1
    unsuitability for pregnant or
        breastfeeding women 171
depression 67, 69, 70
    biogenic amine hypothesis 70–1
    in bipolar disorder 70, 71
    in children and adolescents 141
        treatment 141–4
    co-morbidity with anxiety and
        substance abuse 69, 95, 102
    complementary and alternative
        therapies 78–9, 83
    consumer perspective studies 81–3
    degree of disability with 69
    during breastfeeding, treatment 137
    during pregnancy, treatment 132, 133
    factors influencing recovery from 83
    importance of hope in management of
        82
    and insomnia 107

timing of symptoms following
  commencement of medication 45

fear 95, 98
first generation antipsychotics 4
  adverse effects 4, 43–4, 45, 46, 150–1
  affect on brain structure in
    schizophrenia 43
  affinity for D_2 receptors 43, 45
  for aggression 162
  blocking of central histaminic and
    adrenergic receptors 45–6
  in children and adolescents 140
  combination with SGA 179
  daily dose range 49
  for dementia 58
  during breastfeeding 136
  during pregnancy 131–2
  extrapyramidal side effects 43–4, 45
    detection and management guidelines
    45
  hormonal imbalance involving
    prolactin secretion 45
  in older people 150–1
  perinatal syndrome from 132
  pharmacology 42–6
  for PRN administration 168
  tools for assessing side effects 46
  weight gain associated with 176
'floppy baby' syndrome 132
flumazenil 118
  adverse effects 118
flunitrazepam 106
fluoxetine 4, 75, 137
  for children with OCD 142
  for depression in adolescents 142
  not recommended for older persons 150
fluphenazine 151, 170
fluvoxamine 75, 137
frontal cortex 56
frontal lobes 21

G-protein coupled receptors 116
GABA (gamma-aminobutyric acid) 24, 25
GABA transmitter system, anti-seizure
  agents action on 86
$GABA_A$ receptor complex,
  benzodiazepines action on 101
GABAergic neurotransmission,
  alterations in anxiety disorders 98
gabapentin 98
galactorrhoea 45
galantamine 59, 151

gamma-aminobutyric acid *see* GABA
gastrointestinal tract, factors influencing
  drug absorption 27
general practitioners
  role in management of depression 83
  roles in prescribing psychotropics 11
generalised anxiety disorder 95, 96
  buspirone for 102
genetic factors
  in ADHD 144
  in schizophrenia 42
genetic predisposition, Alzheimer's
  dementia 57–8
glutamate 24, 25
glutametergic transmission, reduction in
  118–19
'Golden Age' of psychopharmacology 4
gynaecomastia 45

hallucinations 39
hallucinogen withdrawal, features 117
hallucinogens 112
haloperidol 151, 162, 163, 168, 170
Hamilton Anxiety Scale (HAMA) 104
health professionals
  attempt to enforce use of psychotropics
    10
  collaboration to provide best outcome
    for consumers 14
  preoccupation with medication to
    detriment of talking and listening
    82
  roles and perspectives on prescribing/
    administration of psychotropics
    10–14
health workers, roles 12–13
hepatic first-pass effects 30
hippocampal neurogenesis 72
hippocampus 55, 67, 72, 73
histaminic receptors, blocking of 45–6, 76
homeostasis 22
Hospital Anxiety and Depression Scale
  (HADS) 104
human rights with regard to
  psychotropic medications 8
5-hydroxytryptamine (5-HT) 24, 25, 70
  receptor sub-types 47
hyperprolactinaemia 45
hypersomnia 105
hypnotics
  benzodiazepine *see* benzodiazepines
  non-benzodiazepine 107
  use in children and young people 107